Group Psychotherapy
for People with Chronic
Mental Illness

Group Psychotherapy for People with Chronic Mental Illness

WALTER N. STONE

The Guilford Press
New York London

Printed in the United States of America

This book is printed on acid-free paper.

Last digit is print number: 9   8   7   6   5   4   3   2   1

Library of Congress Cataloging-in-Publication Data
Stone, Walter N.
    Group Psychotherapy for people with chronic mental illness / Walter N. Stone
        p. cm.
    Includes bibliographical references and index.
    ISBN 1-57230-076-0
    1. Mentally ill—Rehabilitation. 2. Group Psychotherapy.
3. Chronically ill—Rehabilitation. 4. Mentally ill—Social networks.
5. Chronically ill—Social networks. I. Title.
    [DNLM: 1. Psychotherapy, Group. 2. Mental Disorders—therapy.
WM 430 S881g 1996]
RC480.53.S76 1996
616.89'152—dc20
DNLM/DLC
for Library of Congress   95-41586
                                                                    CIP

To my wife,
Esther G. Stone

PREFACE

I t has been my goal in writing this book to provide a coherent dynamic basis for conducting group therapy for chronically mentally ill persons. There is little need to reiterate the plea to find effective interventions to serve this population, which has often been neglected or underserved.

The ascendancy of the biopsychosocial intervention model seems to have been helpful in trying to integrate these dimensions into research and treatment of the chronically ill, but I believe that the psychological dimension has been relatively neglected (if not abandoned) in many settings. Certainly advances continue as technology improves and we are able to make more careful and detailed observations about brain function and biochemical interactions *in situ*. Rehabilitation efforts have also continued in a fashion that has proven helpful to segments of the population. However, the combination of biological elements and interpersonal transactions, often going on for many years, have left emotional scars and sensitivities that cannot be readily altered or eliminated with medication.

A schizophrenic adult, who because of peculiarities as a child was shunned or ridiculed and as a consequence did not develop the interpersonal relationships either inside or outside of the family that might sustain or support him or her, will not have problems solved with medications, even those that hold promise to improve negative symptoms of the illness.

Schizophrenia has been the most extensively studied chronic illness, but other individuals suffering with a variety of disorders, including bipolar illness, major depression or dysthymia, and many persons with Axis II diagnoses become chronically and severely impaired with their illness. There is less research into the problems and habilitation or rehabilitation of these persons, but they are present in every clinic and private population.

Group therapy has the potential of filling many of the needs for patients, but in particular to fulfill their social needs, however limited in comparison to optimal standards. But group treatment is much more than that. It can be, and although the word is out of fashion, should be a place where efforts are made to understand and to remove interferences to successful and satisfying personal relationships.

That is a tall order. There has been an absence of a monograph that would provide clinicians with the historical perspective and the theoretical background to set the stage for group work for the chronically mentally ill. Moreover, integration of dynamic theory and technique in conducting a supportive group treatment that can support individuals in their efforts to stabilize and then change in the direction of improved interpersonal transactions has been missing.

A dynamic approach goes beyond transactions and tries to help individuals modify or heal old internal wounds, thereby gaining new capacities, in essence to become unstuck and restart growth. This is neither simple nor easily accomplished. Patients' many years of caution and fears are not going to dissolve rapidly. Indeed, a hallmark of working with the chronically ill is patience. Elie Wiesel has so sensitively expressed this attribute in his novel *The Fifth Son* (1991), in which he describes the thoughts of a son trying to emotionally contact his father, a concentration camp survivor.

> I also told myself: this is how he is. Nothing I can do about it. Out of reach. I shall have to wait some more. Respect his freedom. Like everyone, he is free to do as he pleases with his past. Free to be a prisoner or a sovereign, resigned or rebellious, friend of the dead or ally of the living. Free to renounce his freedom. I had better accept that. (p. 9)

Time is a precious element. In today's culture trumpeting delivery of services in a rapid and effective manner, working with the chronically ill population stands out as an anomaly. Change does not come about rapidly, and for some, years if not a lifetime of treatment may be necessary. Diabetes, arthritis, cardiac diseases, to name several, are chronic illnesses which medical science is not expected to cure. Rather the clinician's life-time goals are stabilization, prevention of deterioration, and, optimally, relative improvement. Although there may not be precisely defined, societal, wished for biological basis for many mental illnesses, the suffering and disability for the individuals, their family, and those in their social network is at least equal to those with chronic medical illness.

Of course, the clinician does more than wait. It is my hope that this book will provide a clinically salient roadmap in that journey to assist chronically ill persons along the road to more fulfilling and satisfying lives.

ACKNOWLEDGMENTS

I n the process of writing this book, leading, supervising and teaching about groups for chronically ill, I have had an opportunity to reflect upon all of those who have helped me along the way.

One must start with the patients, who have taught me a great deal. However, there is one special group: the members who have consented to having their sessions videotaped and used for educational purposes. I have benefitted enormously from the opportunity they have provided with their generosity. They will remain anonymous, but their contribution I would like duly noted.

I would like to mention a special group of clinicians, the nurses, who have assumed responsibilities for coleading groups with psychiatric residents: Maureen Newlin, Linda Homan, Barbara Wincik, and Molly Cassady. They have taught me a lot as I have conducted supervisory sessions. Special recognition goes to a fifth member of this group, Diana McIntosh, who not only has served as a group leader, but also as Administrator of the Supportive Treatment Service of Central Clinic where these groups have prospered.

I would be remiss not to mention the numerous colleagues in the Department of Psychiatry at the University of Cincinnati College of Medicine who have served as my teachers and mentors. The department was graced by the respect for each person's humanity expressed by Maurice Levine, M.D., the departmental chairman, during my training and early years as a junior faculty member. I hope that my work embodies his oft repeated phrase of "searching for the good inner layer."

My good friend Robert L. Kunkel, M.D., has listened to me discuss my work for many years. His ability to help me understand my group work has proven invaluable.

Howard Kibel, M.D., and Larry Kennedy, M.D., my two friends and colleagues from the American Group Psychotherapy Association, read and commented upon early drafts of this manuscript. I have duly integrated their most helpful suggestions into the final version. Michele Dick valuably assisted in editing many revisions of the manuscript.

One additional group of colleagues also deserves special note: the group of group therapy supervisors who have listened to me present my ideas and case material over an extended period of time. I have grown within their network of intellectual and emotional stimulation: Edward B. Klein, Ph.D; Diana McIntosh, M.S.N.; Janet Newman, M.D.; W. Donald Ross, M.D.; and Murray E. Tieger, Ph.D.

Finally, I would like to thank the sixth member of this group, to whom this book is dedicated, my wife, Esther G. Stone, M.S.S.W., my best critic who has faithfully listened to my efforts to think and write clearly and has provided support and helpful suggestions throughout this entire enterprise.

CONTENTS

Group Psychotherapy
for People with Chronic
Mental Illness

ONE

INTRODUCTION

The inescapable presence of the mentally ill has always raised important issues. What is society's obligation toward them? What is the most effective way of meeting their varied needs? . . . Public policies have often blended such contradictory elements as compassion, sympathy, rejection, and stigmatization. In like vein, psychiatrists have vacillated between emphasizing curability and chronicity; between extreme optimism and a more fatalistic pessimism, and between a commitment to deal with the severely mentally ill and a search to find other kinds of patients.

—GROB (1994, p. 3)

This is a book about the group treatment for the chronically mentally ill. It is based on over two decades of conducting and supervising groups composed of individuals who have been considered unlikely candidates for insight-oriented, self-reflective, individual or group treatment of the kind that is usually highly valued in training centers and in most mental health centers. These are individuals who suffer from multiple disabilities and disadvantages and generally are unable to sustain themselves independently. They do not fulfill the usual role expectations of the culture, either as students, employees, or homemakers. Public funding, with its vagaries and inconsistencies in response to governmental programs and the state of the general economy, is their major source of income.

The continuing seriously mentally ill are at a considerable political disadvantage, and their voices are not readily heard in the chambers of lawmakers or in committee caucuses. Nevertheless, following deinstitu-

1

tionalization there have been some developments in which coordination and continuity of care are provided. The case manager system has the potential for assisting in the multiplicity of needs and providing for continuity, but the danger lurks that this piece of progress will be seen as a substitute for additional therapeutic intervention. Entitlements provide for survival needs, including housing, food, transportation, and general medical care, which are more highly prioritized than patients' emotional needs. Of course, in most instances, medications controlling major symptoms are readily supplied, but pharmacotherapy does not substitute or substantially alter disturbed and disturbing personal relationships that are so frequently a concomitant or intrinsic part of the illness.

The people who are described as continuing and seriously mentally ill are an extremely heterogeneous group, and many of them do not avail themselves of treatment or continuing contact in clinic settings, such as the groups described in this book. Many of those who do come to clinics for treatment merely want medication. Those who do wish for more human contact have had many unsatisfactory or harmful life experiences, and they protect themselves, because they anticipate having their hopes dashed again. One common pattern is to utilize emergency rooms or only intermittently appear for clinic appointments. Others enroll and attend clinics quite regularly if they are not too disturbed or disturbing, but with the typical pressure clinics face to make appointment time available, their appointments will be spaced at greater intervals. The net result is decreasing contact and support, which if sustained at higher levels might have made their lives more satisfactory.

The use of groups in the treatment of these patients arose from several sources. Some patients who had participated in groups during periods of hospitalization continued in groups in the outpatient setting. Other groups arose as an extension of medication clinics where patients were seen for 10- to 15-minute appointments. Observers noted that many patients socialized spontaneously in waiting areas, in contrast to patients' interactions with their physicians in the privacy of the consulting office. These observations stimulated the development of more formal arrangements in which time was allocated for group interaction.

Group structures paralleled individual arrangements. One form primarily focused on provision of medication and socialization among patients was incidental; another form encouraged patients to explore their social relationships and inner experiences. Optimally, this investigation could proceed because patients would provide support for one another, and continuity would be more assured, particularly in training settings, where clinicians would depart at the completion of educational requirements.

These arrangements were not always greeted enthusiastically by clinicians. Some were pleased to have limited contact with patients who erected significant barriers to therapist satisfaction, either because they interacted in a confusing or discomfiting manner or because they responded poorly to treatment. Other therapists, challenged by the difficulties patients presented, were dissatisfied with the limited contact. They believed that more intensive treatment would enable patients to function better, and they suggested a change in the treatment format.

Despite a modicum of enthusiasm for working with groups, many therapists hesitated in assuming leadership responsibilities for groups of persistently and severely mentally ill. In this context, attention shifted to administrative contributions to success and failure of group programs. Dixon (1979), tracing some of the tragedies of British warfare, has explored the psychology of the leadership. He comments, "On logical if not humanitarian grounds the maintenance of an efficient force should be the first consideration of a military commander. Other qualities of generalship will avail him nothing if he has no one left to do the fighting" (p. 153). Similarly, administrators must attend to the needs of therapists, and if support is not available, clinicians often are unwilling to persist in fighting the battles necessary to assist severely ill individuals.

Success in establishing and maintaining a program follows from the happy confluence of an administrator and therapist's empathy for one another's position. Working under the pressures of conducting groups, clinicians often forget that even effective administrators are subjected to many stressors from funding sources and governmental regulations. Many onerous tasks in completing seemingly endless clinical forms and reports are not products of administrative sadism, but are requirements imposed from outside forces. The antidote to staff burnout and abandoning their work is continued administration and clinician collaboration in addressing knotty problems.

The treatment of this population, whatever form is necessary, has to take into account the larger social context and the attributes of the specific setting. Therapists' attention to and efforts at maintaining complex relationships not only with their patients but also within the system will go a long way toward increasing the likelihood of success. The reward for patients and therapists is certainly worthwhile.

This book will address in greater detail the issues introduced here and present many of the theoretical and practical elements necessary to create and sustain an effective and satisfying group treatment program for this significantly underserved population.

TWO

DEFINING CHRONIC
MENTAL ILLNESS

Service systems and the care givers who work in them
must remember that they are responsible for the entire
spectrum of chronic patients, from the least to the most
disabled as well as from those who show promise of
successful rehabilitation to those whose course seems
only to worsen no matter what treatments they receive.

—BACHRACH & LAMB (1989, p. 15)

THE SCOPE OF CHRONIC MENTAL ILLNESS

The equation of chronic mental illness with residence in a state mental hospital and a diagnosis of schizophrenia or major affective disorder has gradually been dispelled. In its place, the boundaries defining chronic mental illness have become blurred. It has not been simple to arrive at a definition delimiting this population.

The "chronically mentally ill population" has been defined as one that "encompasses persons who suffer severe and persistent mental or emotional disorders that interfere with their functional capacities in relation to such primary aspects of daily life as self-care, interpersonal relationships, and work or schooling and that often necessitate prolonged hospital care" (Goldman et al., 1981, p. 22). A later modification of this definition removes the mention of prolonged hospitalization, and focuses more on the individual's "functional capacities in relation to three or more primary aspects of daily life—personal hygiene and self-care, self-direction, interpersonal relationships, social transactions, learning and recreation—that erode or prevent the development of their economic self-sufficiency" (Goldman et al., 1981, p. 23). These criteria are sufficiently broad

4

to include persons who have never been formally diagnosed or received treatment for their symptoms.

Bachrach (1988) remarks about the necessity of clarifying the differences between diagnosis and disability in establishing chronicity. Moreover, she observes that there is no consensus regarding the nature of the interrelationships between three elements—diagnosis, duration, and disability (the three D's)—that have gained acceptance as the basis for defining chronic mental illness.

A similar difficulty exists in defining "chronicity" for medical conditions, as exists for persons with mental illness. Diabetes mellitus is a commonly used illustration of a chronic illness. The diagnosis does not signify the degree of disability, which may range from the minimal need to control one's diet to severe impairment associated with neuropathies and complications of atherosclerosis. A psychiatric diagnosis is necessary but insufficient to carry with it the stigma of chronic illness. For example, patients with bipolar illness may have a manic episode followed by a period of years before a recurrence takes place. They may not necessarily require medication in the interim, and like the diabetic, a recurrence may signal progression of the disease and increasing dysfunction in social relationships and increasing disability in work performance.

The Extent of the Problem

Just as the definition of what constitutes chronic mental illness is elusive, so is the extent of the problem. In the past, it was relatively simple to equate the census in the state hospital system with chronicity, but deinstitutionalization has led to dispersion of many individuals who would have been confined to the hospital. They may live with their families, in welfare hotels, room-and-board homes, independently, or be homeless. The shift in residence from one public-supported facility to another has been labeled "transinstitutionalization."

Goldman et al. (1981) provide information regarding the changing site of patient residence during the most active transitional period of deinstitutionalization. In the quarter of a century between 1955 to 1980, the year-end population of state hospitals in the United States decreased by over 400,000 patients—from a high mark of 559,000 in 1955 to 138,000 in 1980. Bachrach (1992, p. 457) reports unpublished estimates from the National Institute of Mental Health that the 1992 daily state hospital population was about 103,000 patients. In the decade of the 1970s, state hospital admissions decreased from 475,000 to 398,000. These numbers were closely paralleled by a decrease in discharges (501,000 to 395,000). Additionally, the annual hospital death rates in the decade fell from 27,000 to 7,000.

Accompanying these changes was the closing of state hospitals and a loss in available beds. Blaustein (1985) cites the dramatic changes in California, where the population increased from 16 to 25 million from 1960 to 1984, and during the same period, the number of state hospital beds decreased from 37,000 to 5,000. A similar problem of bed shortage was reported in 1980 at the R. H. Hutchings Psychiatric Center in Syracuse, New York, which had a catchment area of 770,000, with only 150 acute care psychiatric beds. Problems of disposition were considerable in the absence of a chronic facility, and community placement was the only available option (Sheets et al., 1982).

In the period 1975–1977, it was estimated that the number of chronically mentally ill ranged from 1.5 to 1.7 million persons (Goldman et al., 1981). About 900,000 of these were institutionalized—150,000 in mental health facilities, 350,000 with mental disorders in nursing homes, and another 400,000 diagnosed as senile in nursing homes. The remaining 700,000 patients were in the community, with about one-half living with relatives, one-fourth living alone, and the remainder in halfway houses, board and care homes, hotels, with friends, or in unknown places.

Counting the mentally ill among the homeless also has been problematic, in part due to the absence of a working definition of homeless, and in part because of the fluctuating nature and diversity of the homeless population (Bachrach, 1992). In 1983 the Alcohol, Drug Abuse and Mental Health Administration estimated about 2 million homeless, of whom one-half were considered to be suffering from drug- or alcohol-related problems or mental illness. The following year, the U.S. Department of Housing and Urban Development estimated the homeless population at between 250,000 and 350,000 persons. Both estimates were found to be flawed (U.S. General Accounting Office, 1988) and no further national estimates have been issued. Estimates of homeless mentally ill persons range from 5% to 90% depending on the site of the survey (Bachrach, 1992, p. 457). Overall, the current judgments are that between one-third and one-half of the homeless are mentally ill. From a different perspective, it is estimated that 5% of severely mentally ill individuals are homeless (Leshner, 1992).

Another subpopulation for whom it is difficult to draw a clear boundary is young adult chronic patients. Many persistently dysfunctional young adults may never be admitted to the state hospital system; instead, they float through the treatment system, using facilities sporadically or inappropriately (Pepper et al., 1981). The diagnostic spectrum of those individuals is varied and includes psychosis and personality disorders, often complicated by substance abuse. Characteristic of this subgroup are the members' severe social, vocational, and mental impairment.

With this brief review of the scope of the problem, the model proposed by Bachrach (1988) elucidating the three major dimensions of chronic mental illness—diagnosis, disability, and duration—will be examined in more detail.

DIAGNOSIS

Schizophrenia

Beginning with the integrative work of Bleuler (1911), the schizophrenias were assumed to have a progressively deteriorating course, ending in dementia. Yet, even in Bleuler's initial study, about 15% of persons diagnosed with this illness were found to recover. Introduction of modern psychopharmacology did not appear to greatly alter the course of the disease, although the positive symptoms (hallucinations, delusions, thought disorganization, etc.) were brought under improved control.

McGlashan (1988) reviewed the long-term outcome studies of schizophrenia during the preceding quarter of a century. His stringent selection criteria limited the scope of the review to 10 studies or groups of studies. "Long-term" was defined as a minimum average of 10 years. Overall, the findings confirmed the observation by Bleuler that schizophrenia is a chronic illness that frequently disables for a lifetime, and the average outcome is worse than that of other major mental illnesses.

Fifty percent of young adult schizophrenic patients have poor global outcomes, characterized by severe impairment due to symptoms, poor social functioning, or suicide (Breier et al., 1991; Carone et al., 1991). Indeed, contributing to the morbidity and mortality of schizophrenia is the increased risk for suicide and physical illness (Black, 1988).

Rehospitalization was found to decrease across a 5-year period (Carone et al., 1991), and with adequate treatment, positive symptoms may level off, whereas negative symptoms may increase and are correlated with social functioning (Breier et al., 1991).

Socioeconomic factors appear to influence global outcome. Patients living in the inner city fare more poorly than those in rural settings, where conditions may be more similar to Third World countries and the course of the illness is more benign (World Health Organization, 1979). Patients discharged in rural circumstances may reach a plateau in the second to third decade of illness (Harding et al., 1987a, 1987b). McGlashan (1988, p. 529), accounting for differences in outcome between studies of patients from the Boston State Hospital and Chestnut Lodge, speculated that the economic resources may improve living situations and employment opportunities. The degree of remaining psychopathology was not similarly influenced.

Changes in outcome may reflect changes in diagnostic criteria. Reflecting the narrow definition of schizophrenia reintroduced with the third edition of the *Diagnostic and Statistical Manual of Mental Disorders* (DSM-III; American Psychiatric Association, 1980), a large-scale review of outcome studies found the proportion of patients rated improved in the period 1956–1985 to be 48.5%, and improvement rates were 36.4% in the succeeding decade, which closely approximated the 35.4% level found in the period 1895–1955 (Hegarty et al., 1994). Psychosocial factors may influence a person's living situation and perhaps his or her social relationships, but as summarized by McGlashan (1988), "Long-term follow-up studies have yet to demonstrate clearly any effect of treatment on the natural history of schizophrenia" (p. 515).

Schizoaffective Disorders

The diagnosis of schizoaffective disorder has commanded a place on the boundary between affective and schizophrenic illnesses and has presented nosological problems (Coryell et al., 1990). Schizoaffective individuals were found to have somewhat poorer functioning than patients with bipolar manic illness and considerably poorer functioning that patients with unipolar disorder. They fared better, however, than the comparison schizophrenic patients (Grossman et al., 1991; Keller et al., 1986a). Outcome appears to be more linked with psychotic-like symptoms than affective syndromes (Grossman et al., 1991).

Mood Disorders

Mania

The impact of effective antimanic treatments has not impacted upon the outcome of bipolar affective disorder as greatly as originally hoped. Lithium, hailed as a specific chemotherapeutic treatment, has failed to live up to initial expectations. Only about 20% of manic patients treated with lithium will have no further episodes of illness. The remaining patients will have one or more recurrences, which are associated with progressive deterioration in functioning (Prien & Gelenberg, 1989). Even before they recover from their index episode of mania, 15–30% will cycle into depression (Tohen et al., 1990; Keller et al., 1986b). Moreover, rapid cyclers are notoriously poor responders to a variety of medication regimens. Mixed or dysphoric states, which are characterized by mania or hypomania concomitant with major depressive symptoms, may be present in 30–40% of manic episodes. Response to treatment appears less certain than in simple mania (Swann, 1995). Further contributing to the pool of chronic patients are individuals who present management problems such as medication noncompliance, concomitant medical illnesses, substantial impairment in interepisode functioning, and substance abuse (Prien & Gelenberg, 1989, p. 841). Newer antimanic medications, carbamazepine and valproate, have produced better improvement rates, but the disability associated with manic illness remains substantial.

Depression

Depressive disorders are chronic illnesses with more than 50% recurrence rates (Keller & Hanks, 1994). Major depressive syndromes are associated with considerable morbidity and mortality (approximately 15% of patients with major depression commit suicide; Guze & Robins, 1970). Mood-incongruent outcome resembles that of mood-congruent depression and is dissimilar to the poorer prognosis of schizophrenic and schizoaffective disorders (Tsuang & Coryell, 1993). Delusions and hallucinations coexisting with mood disorders tend to inhibit recovery (Dubovsky & Thomas, 1992). An initial, good treatment response is not always maintained (Aronson et al., 1988), but over extended periods, psychotically depressed patients have outcomes similar to those with nonpsychotic depression (Coryell & Tsuang, 1982).

Depressive symptoms of insufficient duration or intensity may be present prior to the onset of a diagnosable major affective illness, which then may be diagnosed double depression (Horwath et al., 1992; Wells et al., 1992); however, treatment may lead to resolution in only 65–80% of individuals (Baldessarini, 1989), and 12% may not have recovered in 5 years (Keller et al., 1992). Initial symptom severity, earlier age of onset, and a family history of depressive illness are predictors of outcome (Warner et al., 1992). Incomplete resolution of a major depression may by evidenced by symptoms of sufficient intensity to qualify for a diagnosis of dysthymia, which in itself accounts for considerable morbidity.

A more optimistic series of reports suggest that high maintenance dosage of antidepressants (200 mg of imipramine) and monthly interpersonal therapy are successful in preventing relapse (Frank et al., 1990; Kupfer et al., 1992). However, troublesome side effects interfere with patient compliance with traditional tricyclic medications. The newer selective serotonin reuptake inhibitors (SSRIs) are found to be as efficacious as tricyclic antidepressants for severe depression, although data for inpatients are limited (Nierenberg, 1994).

Depression is a recurrent and a chronic illness, and the nature of impairment in work, family relations, and social adjustment is not inconsequential, with high rates of disability concomitant and welfare assistance (Klerman & Weissman, 1992; Coryell et al., 1993).

Anxiety Disorders

Anxiety disorders, which cover a broad range of symptoms, are often associated with chronicity. Patients with generalized anxiety disorder (GAD) may be symptomatic for many years and only partially responsive to pharmacological treatment. Their quality of life may be significantly impaired. Relapses, which occur at variable intervals following discontinuation of medications, are not uncommon for this group of patients (Gorman & Papp, 1990). Patients with GAD have been found to have other anxiety disorders or major depression (Massion et al., 1993). Of patients with panic attacks, 75–90% can become symptom free with medication (Fyer & Sandberg, 1988). Pharmacotherapy, however, does not effectively treat worry about panic or avoidant (agoraphobic) behaviors that require additional treatment interventions (Fyer & Sandberg, 1988, p. 115). Severe obsessive–compulsive disorders are particularly disabling. Newer medications have been of significant help in combating the major symptoms, but a portion of obsessive patients remains symptomatic and disabled.

Added to the list of anxiety disorders is posttraumatic stress disorder, which is often severe and disabling.

Many patients with anxiety disorders have associated Axis II diagnoses. The outcome of pharmacotherapy is diminished and psychotherapeutic efforts may also fail, a situation that further contributes to the pool of chronically ill individuals.

Substance Abuse

The prevalence of substance abuse among the chronically mentally ill is substantial. Rates may range from 25% to 75% in the reported surveys (Bergman & Harris, 1985; Court et al., 1971; Safer, 1987; Test et al., 1985). Patients with dual diagnoses (substance abuse and mental illness) more often are male, younger, and socially disorganized with respect to maintenance of housing, finances, and food. They clinically showed greater hostility, suicidality, and speech disorganization, and had poorer medication compliance (Drake & Wallach, 1989, p. 1041). The latter behaviors are believed to represent disinhibition rather than specific increased psychotic symptoms (p. 1044).

Caton et al. (1989), in a study of a long-term cohort of young adults and adolescents, report that 51% had a dual diagnosis and more than two-thirds of those individuals did not use drugs until after the onset of their psychiatric illness. Polydrug use was present in one-half of the drug-using population. The diagnosis of substance abuse is not simple. In a study of patients referred to a state hospital from a psychiatric emergency room, only a small number of drugs was detected in the emergency room. The extent of the drug usage was found to be greater at the time of admission, and an almost fivefold increase in drug usage was detected when a research team assessed patients when they had sufficiently recovered from the acute phase of their illness to cooperate in providing a more detailed history (Ananth et al., 1989).

The interrelationship between chronic mental illness and substance abuse remains to be clarified. Minkoff (1989), representing one position, supports the notion of a parallel disease model for chronic mental illness and substance abuse: "In each model the illness or disease is an incurable, biologic mental disorder, most commonly characterized by a chronic course with multiple relapses and exacerbations. Even though symptoms may remit for long periods, the potential for relapse is generally always present" (p. 1032).

Personality Disorders

Patients with DSM-IV Axis II disorders also contribute to the pool of the chronically mentally ill. The three clusters of personality disorders have characteristics that may be sufficiently prominent in the individual's presentation to lead to enduring work and social disability. The characterization of odd and eccentric behaviors for "Cluster A" (paranoid, schizoid, and schizotypal personality disorders), frequent dramatic, emotional behaviors for "Cluster B" (antisocial, borderline, histrionic, and narcissistic personality disorders), and anxious fearfulness for "Cluster C" (avoidant, dependent, and obsessive–compulsive disorders) speaks to the patients' difficulties (American Psychiatric Association, 1994).

Reich and Green (1991) reviewed the effect of personality disorders on the treatment outcome of Axis I diagnoses. Despite methodological limitations, including the absence of "blind" raters, the data were described as robust, confirming that patients with personality pathology have poorer treatment response than those individuals without such diagnoses. The authors observed that studies using standardized measure of personality disorder may be confounded by Axis II symptoms confusing and intensifying Axis I symptoms. Outcomes of specific Axis I disorders that were negatively affected were major depression, panic disorder, and obsessive–compulsive disorder. The comorbidity of depression with personality disorder was found, following treatment, to lead to greater maladjustment in social functioning, but not in work functioning. Moreover, patients were less likely to reach criteria for symptomatic recovery (Shea et al., 1990).

DURATION

The very concept of chronicity implies long-term impairments. Duration includes both past and future behavior. The term itself has been under attack because of concern over the impact of labeling, which may lead to self-fulfilling prophecy either on the part of the patient or through the impact on the environment. Duration is intimately linked with disability, more so in terms of fulfilling social roles and expectations rather than specific symptoms. By the time some persons first come to the attention of mental health professionals, they can be determined to have been disabled for an extended period. Careful history will reveal a failure to reach age-appropriate functions or a gradual decline of functions that had been achieved.

A rapid onset of an initial illness is considered a prognosticator of good recovery, but many mental illnesses are characterized by relapsing states, even with optimal available treatment. Each recurrence decreases the likelihood of regaining previously established functional capacities. The course of an illness leading to chronicity is multidimensional.

The time period defining chronicity usually coincides with requirements for entitlements. For instance, Social Security Administration (SSA) cutoffs for chronic schizophrenia require a documented history of one or more clearly defined episodes that include symptom pictures and functional limitations. In addition, requirements include functional deterioration following major symptom recurrence or a documented history of 2 or more years of inability to function outside a supportive living situation.

The interaction between the time conundrum and functional capacity serves to maintain chronicity in a portion of this population. Many patients might be able to work. Liberalization of rules allowing a disabled person to work full time for a specified period (e.g., 6–9 months) before giving up entitlements has had some adherents. However, the available positions are usually for low pay with minimal or no benefits. The trade-off gain of an enhanced self-esteem attendant with employment appears to be unbalanced when compared with the loss of entitlements.

· DISABILITY

Equally as problematic as establishing diagnosis and duration in defining chronic mental illness is establishing criteria for disability. The political rhetoric about welfare and Social Security disability abusers is ample evidence of the emotional response of the general public to the "disabled" and the lack of consistently applicable operational criteria defining disability.

"Disability," broadly considered, is the inability to fulfill reasonable societal expectations of work and social activities. Those functions are partially independent of specific psychiatric diagnoses. Gruenberg (1967) separated the components of disability into those arising from the individual's capacities and those arising from social expectations. The patient's contribution may arise from the specific symptoms of the illness and the experience of the illness itself. This would include responses such as inhibitions or anxiety about the recurrence of the illness. Societal contributions include stigmatization, diminished social networks, poverty, unemployment, and a general lack of belonging (Bachrach, 1986, p. 981).

Transcultural studies have demonstrated different frequencies of mental illness, social disability, and symptoms in different cultures (Leff, 1988). Social support and acceptance of "deviance" permit the individual with some impairment to remain in and be a productive member of the culture. In a U.S. study, Davies et al. (1989) assessed the adjustment of schizophrenic patients living in urban and rural settings. Based on the patients' self-reports, individuals living in the city had greater psychopathology and poorer social adjustment, quality of life, and global functioning. The authors attribute the differences to the higher levels of stress in the urban setting, where "neighborhoods are more likely to be aversive, living situations are more likely to be conflictual, and patients are less likely to receive practical support from home operators. These conditions may overtax already vulnerable individuals, thus engendering social withdrawal and isolation" (p. 829).

Employment rates are significantly diminished for patients discharged from psychiatric hospitals. The person's ability to find work and then maintain him- or herself on the job is substantially impaired (Jacobs et al., 1992). More than two-thirds of individuals with chronic mental illness remain unemployed (Goldstrom & Mandersheid, 1972). Anthony and Jansen (1984) reviewed the literature predicting patients' vocational capacities. Among their findings were the relative independence of psychiatric symptomatology and diagnosis from work capacity. A person's ability to function in one setting was not predictive of ability to function in another. However, an individual's ability to "get along" or function socially with others was found to be a significant predictor of future work performance.

Impaired social functioning is one component in determining eligibility for disability benefits. An individual's capacity to form and sustain mutually supportive relationships is subject to a variety of measurements.

Clarity of communication that may include both verbal and nonverbal elements, willingness to receive and offer help to others, and the more obvious capacity to get along in the workplace with coworkers or supervisors, or difficulties with the law, are some of the components that are evaluated in social functioning.

Disability also is based on an individual's capacity to independently maintain activities of daily living. The ability to care for one's residence, arrange and prepare meals, use transportation, and pay bills is part of the global assessment in this sector. Added to these criteria are the person's capacity to maintain appropriate grooming and hygiene. The overlap between social relationships and independent living skills is not insignificant.

An often overlooked element in the chronic patient's disability is the increased likelihood of a concurrent medical illness. In one study, more then 50% of chronic psychiatric patients were found to have chronic medical problems that interfered with their daily lives (McCarrick et al., 1986) The percentages vary across studies (Koranyi, 1979; Barnes et al., 1983) but many of the illnesses are undiagnosed. Roca et al. (1987), in a sample of 42 patients in a psychosocial rehabilitation program, found that 93% of the individuals had at least one problem that warranted assessment. Minor gynecological disease was the most common problem among women, and gross dental problems were most common among men. Only 11% of the men's problems and 26% of the women's problems were receiving appropriate care. An expanded study of 195 homeless persons (not all of whom were mentally ill) reported similar results. Men were found to have an average of 8.3 problems, and women to have 9.2 problems (Breakey et al., 1989).

An operational basis for defining disability often is based on eligibility for existing government entitlement programs, such as the Federal Supplemental Security Income (SSI) Program. Historically, eligibility criteria were based primarily on prior hospitalization, despite the fact that many of the disabled younger adults had never been hospitalized.

State-to-state variation in eligibility requirements is considerable. A particularly salient study was conducted by Schinnar et al. (1990). Definitions of chronic mental illness used in 10 states[1] were applied to a sample of 222 patients, including 60% Medicaid recipients, admitted to an inner-city mental health center. Forty-one percent of those individuals received SSI or Social Security Disability Insurance (SSDI) benefits. Using the different definitions, the prevalence estimates of patients defined as chronically mentally ill ranged from 38% to 72%. The National Institute of Mental Health definition yielded a prevalence of 55%. Thus the national estimates of the prevalence of chronic mental illness are at best a rough estimate of the actual numbers.

SUMMARY

Defining and delimiting the chronically mentally ill population have been fraught with problems. Limiting the definition to particular diagnoses has not been helpful, because a wide range of functional impairment may be associated with all of the diagnoses. In great measure, the problem is sociopolitical. Certainly chronically mentally ill individuals with limited political power are subject to political pressures that redefine the boundaries of eligibility based on bias and fiscal restraints. The functional definition at one time may not be applicable at another. Bachrach's (1988) lament, "Despite growing recognition of its irrelevance, the criterion of prior hospitalization remains a strong official and de facto indicator of chronicity in many jurisdictions" (p. 385), is but one example of the failure of the political system to keep pace with social changes.

A great deal of research is necessary to clarify the interaction between the three D's—diagnosis, duration, and disability. The extent of the functional disability of significant duration in persons with a diagnosable mental illness is the most salient definition of the chronically mentally ill population, but there is potential for rehabilitation or improved quality of life for almost all of this population, and the dimensions of their disability remain great.

The relevance of defining the total population of the chronically mentally ill for the group therapist is to place the various group intervention strategies in the broad perspective of the problem of providing service for this population. No single program will serve all.

THREE

HISTORY

*We consider a therapeutic procedure scientifically
founded if it is based on the knowledge of the disease
which it attempts to remedy and on the understanding
of the curative process itself.*

—ALEXANDER (1946, p. 110)

Only slowly has the scientific basis for understanding basic
biopsychosocial dynamics of the chronically mentally ill
emerged. For at least a portion of the schizophrenic and major
affective-disordered individuals, solid evidence of a biologi-
cal/hereditary element exists. Other evidence implicates the role of interpersonal stress as either etiological or precipitating conditions leading to
the eruption of major symptoms. The nature–nurture controversy continues to intrigue clinicians and researchers.

The theoretical and clinical understandings of group and individual
dynamics combined with "practical" needs for both patients and the
therapeutic culture have produced a spectrum of group treatment strategies for the chronically mentally ill. Sophisticated research in this area,
however, has been spotty. Therapists embarking on the task of creating
and sustaining groups for the chronically ill population are dependent on
clinical lore and the limited available research in gaining an overview of
treatment approaches.

This chapter will review the history of outpatient groups for the
chronically ill population.

THE BEGINNINGS

Prior to World War II, the value of group treatment for many mental disorders was being explored. Outpatient groups for the seriously mentally ill arose primarily from efforts to provide treatment for patients discharged from mental hospitals. Gifford and MacKenzie (1948) reviewed the early literature on group treatment of psychoses prior to and following World War II. They described three major approaches to group treatment for this population.

1. Didactic methods, in which lectures based primarily on psychoanalytic concepts were given to educate patients about mental mechanisms. In this model, the therapist encouraged discussion of symptoms, such as delusions or hallucinations, and made an effort to provide patients with an intellectual understanding of their illness. The therapist thus assumed the role of teacher. E. W. Lazell, Louis Wender, and J. W. Klapman were identified as the most influential practitioners of this approach.

2. Repressive–inspirational methods that placed the therapist in the role of an inspirational leader. L. Cody Marsh, the foremost advocate of this method, utilized "whatever therapeutic devices could be usefully adapted from the popular forms of mass psychology, the emotional appeal of the evangelistic revival meeting and the commercial techniques of the business men's luncheons" (p. 22). This approach takes advantage of positive transferences to the leader, and identification among the members to induce change.

3. Traditional analytic methods, which were generally eschewed. However, beginning in the early 1930s, Paul Schilder conducted groups based on analytic principles. For example, patients wrote autobiographies to provide the therapist with historical information that might be utilized for interpretation. Schilder also attempted to elicit dynamic material within the transference and resistance paradigms. He felt that he had efficacious results with schizophrenic but not with depressed patients.

Groups were primarily, but not exclusively hospital based. The advent of World War II and the success in treating military personnel in groups seemed to energize interest in group approaches.

THE EARLY YEARS

The period following the end of the war was one of euphoria, in which the military success and the elevation of the United States to a super-power status was evident in the energy and enthusiasm with which societal problems were tackled. There was a growing interest in psychoanalytic concepts in the field of psychiatry, and for a period, dynamic psychiatry eclipsed biology. Psychoanalytic concepts were applied in social situations. Concepts of the therapeutic community were utilized in hospital settings, and intensive psychotherapeutic treatment of schizophrenic patients was attempted in prestigious hospitals such as the Menninger Foundation, Chestnut Lodge, and the Austin Riggs Center. Even the popular literature reflected the culture, with publication of the best-seller *I Never Promised You a Rose Garden*, which described the psychotherapeutic explorations into the inner world of a schizophrenic girl.

Outpatient groups for the seriously mentally ill in the immediate postwar period, which preceded availability of effective pharmacotherapy, reflected a certain ambivalence. The enthusiasm for psychoanalytic ideas was tempered by concerns that the population, defined primarily as schizophrenia, could not or would not benefit from such treatment. Nevertheless, homogeneous groups were organized for patients provisionally discharged from mental hospitals. Many were time limited, ranging from 6 to 12 months, a duration that coincided with the departure of an interested therapist from training (Polan & Spark, 1950; Blau & Zilbach, 1954). In some instances, however, patients anticipating termination of their group asked that the sessions be continued, and they developed sufficient relatedness and cohesion that they resisted newcomers (Talmadge, 1959).

An alternate approach for a limited segment of the chronically ill population was to include one or two "nonpsychotic" schizophrenic patients in mixed analytic groups (Spotnitz, 1957; Hulse, 1958; Feldberg, 1958). This ill-defined diagnostic grouping contained individuals who were labeled as pseudoneurotic, or as having simple or postpsychotic schizophrenia, and so forth. These patients, at times, aided other group members through their ability to verbalize deep feelings, but they had difficulty utilizing such information for their own benefit.[1]

These early reports revealed practitioners to be surprised and pleased with the manner in which patients were able to form useful group relationships. Experience promoted changes in therapeutic technique, in which interpretative interventions were partially replaced by efforts to promote member interaction (Klapman, 1951; Talmadge, 1959).

EXPANSION

The decade of the 1960s was marked by significant social and political change. The Vietnam War produced major upheavals in the United States. Protests against the government were rampant; social alienation and dropping out were commonplace. One cultural antidote was the emergence of the encounter group movement that promised a pathway to intimacy and countered the alienation of normal people.

The chronically mentally ill were among the most alienated in the society. They had been sequestered in state mental hospitals, but the periodic public outcry about their treatment led to the formation of the Joint Commission on Mental Health, which published its final report, *Action for Mental Health,* in 1961. The report outlined community alternatives to the state hospital. Moreover, the advent of effective medications and a philosophy of social treatment further contributed to the belief that the state mental hospital was *not* an appropriate treatment setting for the great majority of chronic patients (Lamb, 1984). Legislation enacted in 1963 provided categorical Aid to the Disabled (ATD, now called Supplemental Security Income [SSI]) and included the mentally ill. In addition, federal monies became available to construct and staff community mental health centers.

Discharges from mental hospitals accelerated, but the enthusiasm of the movement catapulted patients out of the hospital into the community without sufficient preparation for their care. Readmission rates did not change (Goldman et al., 1981), and a substantial number of seriously mentally ill joined the homeless population (Lamb, 1984).

This milieu spawned an increase in exploration of group treatments for the chronically mentally ill. Reports of lengthy treatment endeavors, ranging from 6 to 10 years, reinforced the belief that patients could beneficially engage in such treatment. Therapeutic formats, however, frequently were altered, and groups met at biweekly or monthly intervals, rather than the traditional weekly sessions. Medication was held out as the initial carrot, a strategy that served to sustain patients' attendance (Janecek & Mandel, 1965; Payne, 1965). Attention was paid to engaging lower socioeconomic level patients into groups by providing prompt access to treatment (Beck, 1969) or by attending to the social context of minority communities (Christmas, 1966).

The boundaries of treatment were altered in a variety of ways. Waiting rooms were seen as places to encourage patient interaction as clinic staff moved out of their offices to promote patient dialogue (Rada et al., 1964; Masnik et al., 1971). Coffee and food served as enticements to patient attendance, a strategy that carried over into the more formal treatment room (Donlon et al., 1973). Relatives were actively engaged and encouraged to inform clinicians of drug side effects when injectable medications were administered as part of the group treatment. The establishment of a monthly parallel group for relatives of schizophrenic patients who attended their own group was associated with decreased use of hospital services (Battegay & Von Marschall, 1978). These strategies not only served to promote interaction among members, but functioned as an additional inducement for patients to attend treatment. Cooper (1978) observed that leverage in the form of legal or family pressure was sometimes necessary to help patients attend or remain in the group. Employing a different strategy to engage patients, MacKenzie (1974) described a home group program in which schizophrenic women met weekly in one another's homes under the supervision of a nurse, who also would drive some members to the meeting.

Efforts to evaluate the effectiveness of the various group programs were beset with multiple difficulties. Comparisons were made between group and individual treatment, and within a group, between use of injectable and oral medications. Differences in frequency of treatment or vague descriptions of the treatment strategies, such as groups that focused primarily on medication compliance, and differences in experience and skill of the clinicians, created difficulties in comparing outcomes across the various studies.

Parloff and Dies (1977), in a review paper, opined:

> "Group psychotherapy" as an undefined treatment form for post-hos-pital schizophrenics does not appear to contribute uniquely or consis-tently to the amelioration of such target treatment areas as reduced rates of rehospitalization, improved vocational adjustment, or diminished psychopathology, or enhanced social effectiveness. It does appear, how-ever, to provide a useful supplement to other psychosocial treatment efforts. (p. 295)[2]

Mosher and Keith (1980), reviewing psychosocial treatments for schizo-phrenic patients, commented that group treatment "whose principal aim is to promote socialization and enhance interpersonal skills should not be expected to have a striking effect on rehospitalization rates or vocational adjustment" (p. 148).

RECENT DECADES

The social climate changed considerably, beginning in the decade of the 1980s. The myth of the 1980s, according to Haynes Johnson (1992), was that

> the United States of America . . . had fallen into a state of disintegration and with Ronald Reagan recaptured what it had lost: optimism; strength; enterprise; inventiveness. Most of all America wanted to believe it had recaptured a sense of success. Success for the nation, success for the individual: In the public mind, the two were indivisible. (p. 13)

Support of social welfare was replaced by an entrepreneurial spirit; each individual could achieve through the dint of his or her own efforts. The publication in 1980 of DSM-III represented a profound shift in American psychiatry. In part, DSM-III was a response to the lack of clarity between health and illness in the biopsychosocial model of illness. Diagnosis shifted to a descriptive psychiatry and "clinicians were replaced by biomedical researchers as the most influential voices in the field" (Wilson, 1993, p. 408). Advances in biological treatments were a consequence of and a stimulus for research monies to be shifted from psychosocial treatment to biological research. Psychiatry declared the 1990s the "decade of the brain."

As a reflection of these trends, few projects assessing outcome of group interventions appeared. Anticipating the emphasis on brief treatment, Kanas and his colleagues (Kanas, 1991; Kanas & Smith, 1990; Kanas et al., 1989a, 1989b) studied 12-week time-limited groups for schizophrenic patients, addressing patients' psychotic experiences, their ways of coping, and their social isolation. Kanas believes that the well-defined goals provided protection for the patients and enabled them to make gains in social and symptomatic spheres. Patients were also enrolled in a medication clinic, where their treatment continued beyond the group experience. In part, the model addressed patients' clinical condition because shortened hospital stays often resulted in their being discharged with incompletely resolved psychotic symptoms. Malm (1982), comparing group and standard treatments, initiated group treatment of 12 months' duration 2 months postdischarge. Measures of social function favored group treatment, but several differences did not appear until 1–2 years after the index admission. Commenting on the Malm study, Keith and Mathews (1984) observed:

> These results highlight the importance of the timing of the initiation of a psychotherapy study: If begun too early (at a time when positive symptoms predominate, and outcome is therefore appropriately measured in terms of symptom remission), most of the variability will be accounted for by the drug effect; if begun too late, there will be little variability left to account for in evaluating the outcome. The optimal time, according to this, would appear to be in the outpatient stabilization period. (p. 79)

The introduction of lithium salts as a primary treatment for manic–depressive patients stimulated interest in groups composed exclusively of those individuals (Vokmar et al., 1981; Kripke & Robinson, 1985; Wulsin et al., 1988; Cerbone et al., 1992). Those preliminary reports were encouraging and suggested that the treatment decreased hospitalization rates and improved social functioning.

Groups formed for individuals with a single diagnosis represented one treatment strategy, as exemplified by individuals diagnosed with bipolar disorder or schizophrenia. The increasing use of clozapine, with its associated stringent requirements for obtaining blood counts, spawned an additional subset of groups.

Alternative strategies became evident in this period, coinciding with the expansion of the definition of the chronically mentally ill. Groups were planned for individuals receiving a variety of both Axis I and Axis II diagnoses. The groups were relatively homogeneous from the perspective of the members' impairment (de Bosset, 1988, 1991; McIntosh et al., 1991). Because communication among schizophrenic members was limited and attendance was variable, the advantages of this strategy were to increase member interaction and provide for greater continuity. Within the broad range of disabilities exhibited in the population, further subgrouping of patients by functional level was attempted (Misunis et al., 1990). Patients' cognitive style may limit gains, and concrete forms of social support and advice giving can be effective therapeutic tools (Weiner, 1988).

Among the strategies designed to maintain group attendance and increase socialization was enlarging the group roster to 12 or more individuals, with the expectation that a number of patients would not attend any particular meeting (McGee, 1983). Other researchers suggested contracting with members in order to set expectations of frequency of attendance (Lesser & Friedmann, 1980; Kimmel, 1991; McIntosh et al., 1991). In this format, individuals would not be expected to attend every meeting, but they would be expected to abide by the attendance agreement that they had negotiated with the therapist. In this model, patients form a core subgroup of regular attenders and a peripheral subgroup of intermittent attenders. Both subgroups are thought to benefit from group participation. Over time, patients may decrease their attendance yet remain linked to treatment, thereby providing cost-effective therapy (Stone, 1995).

Acceptance of patients bringing young children to the group appeared to increase member interaction and enliven the meetings (Stone, 1983). Setting the time of the group in the late morning set the stage for patients to go to lunch together (Seeman, 1981).

As managed care expands to include the public sector, evidence indicates that as few as 12 group sessions in 1 year sharply decrease the number of hospitalization and in-hospital days. Some cost savings may have been shifted to increased attendance at nonpsychiatric clinics (Weiner, 1992).

Attention also was focused on the problem of staff burnout, and structures to support the staff were developed. The strategies included use of cotherapists or alternating leaders (Levin et al., 1985), continuing supervision (McGee, 1983), and postgroup team meetings (de Bosset, 1991). Elucidation of the universal dynamics of therapists' needs for emotional connection with their patients and professional satisfaction helps maintain clinicians' interest in working with this population (Stone, 1991).

SUMMARY

This review of outpatient dynamic psychotherapy groups for the chronically mentally ill has attempted to place this modality in the scientific framework suggested by Alexander (1946). A considerable body of clinical experience has accumulated that attests to the efficacy of this treatment. However, the research, which has generally been favorable, has not been robust. Problems in specifying the type of group, the frequency of attendance, and treatment goals have hampered interpretation of the data. Comparisons of group therapy with other treatments are few. The design of studies that compare individual and group therapy often provides only limited treatment contact and may be more useful in supporting patients' acceptance of their medication than in assisting in the solution of social relationship problems.

Many of the early reports addressed groups composed primarily of patients diagnosed with schizophrenia; considerably less information is available regarding the behavior of the large segment of chronically mentally ill population who have other diagnoses or who have not had extended periods of hospitalization.

Whereas early reports were more focused on the patient's capacity to remain out of hospital (through stabilization of major symptoms), more recent reports focus on the patient's ability to manage in the community and be satisfied with life, as expressed by improved social interaction. Extended treatment periods of more than 1 year may be necessary before improvement in social functioning is observable. However, some evidence has emerged that carefully structured short-term groups can effect change in social relationships.

Recent trends with diagnostically heterogeneous groups seem promising, but with the decrease in outcome studies in the past decade, controlled outcome data are lacking.

Finally, clinicians at all levels of experience working with this population are subject to discouragement, loss of interest, and burnout. There has been a growing emphasis on the need to provide support for therapists, particularly those who may be relatively inexperienced, unfamiliar with the depth of pathology of the chronically mentally ill, and therefore least prepared to handle the stresses of working with this population.

FOUR

THE IMPACT OF SOCIAL RELATIONS ON CHRONIC MENTAL ILLNESS

All human beings, including those who are mentally ill can be influenced by their current environment, particularly when it resonates with important past experiences.

—CANCRO (1983, p. 494)

A person's capacity to develop and maintain relationships is a product of many interacting factors. Biological vulnerabilities or variations may combine with caregivers' or peers' capabilities to empathically interact. The result may either enhance or diminish an individual's capacity to manage stress. Chronically ill patients often suffer with limitations in their social relations. The breadth of their personal networks may be restricted, and the number of those with whom they might have developed intimate associations may be even more limited. The result is that patients may be unable to avail themselves of helpful support in managing their mental illness.

This chapter will review development of social relationships and its role in the recovery from illness.

SOCIAL RELATIONSHIPS IN THE LIFE CYCLE

The developmental achievements of the healthy child depend on the availability of appropriate and responsive interaction with others. De-

24

tailed explorations of early infant behavior have demonstrated that the newborn is capable of responding in a discriminating fashion to evidence of a relationship (Stern, 1985). An infant's capacity to bond and form attachments to others may be a consequence of temperamental differences (Chess & Hassibi, 1986). The unavailability of responsive persons in the first months of life leads to severe developmental retardation (Spitz, 1963).

As the child moves out of the exclusive sphere of the family and begins peer play, the caregiver's ability to provide a holding environment (Winnicott, 1965) is seen as critical. For the growing child, peers take on increasing importance and add to self-esteem. According to Grunebaum and Solomon (1987), "Peers probably promote collaborative problem solving and certainly foster a higher developmental level of play with toys than occurs with adult care givers or when the toddler is alone" (p. 490).

Sullivan (1953) posited that a latency child's social development culminates in the establishment of "chumship" with a same-sex friend. The chum is not a person who is utilized to fulfill the child's own needs but rather one for whom the child develops a genuine sensitivity.

Boys and girls' feelings about relationships diverge. Generally, boys are concerned with achieving and establishing their sense of self through sports and other competitions that are bounded by external rules. Usually, girls are concerned with maintaining relationships expressed in their attachments and sensitivities to the needs of others and will eschew competition rather than disrupt a relationship (Gilligan, 1982).

The biological changes in adolescence are accompanied by development of age-appropriate heterosexual interests and by further efforts to emancipate the adolescent from the family. Optimally, it is the family's understanding of these tasks that allows the adolescent to experiment, knowing that freedom exists within limits.

Social relationships are also of major significance in this era. Being "in" with the peer group is desirable, if not emotionally essential. Fads, such as clothing and hairstyles, are ways of belonging to the peer group and separating from parental values. Those who are not part of the idealized group suffer considerable struggles with self-esteem. Of course, those who are "in" have their own difficulties as they try to maintain their "place in the sun," often in the face of internal uncertainties and doubts. The intrapsychic conflicts stemming from previously established (internalized) family standards contribute to the tumultuous tasks of adolescents.

In the past three decades, increasing attention has been paid to the developmental tasks of adulthood. The contributions of Erikson (1963) place developmental stages in a much clearer social perspective. As symbolic functioning stabilizes and physical maturity is approached, the pace of change diminishes. Michaels (1980) remarks, "Psychological development of the adult results primarily from interaction with experience, integrated in symbolic forms" (p. 26).

Different models for understanding adult development have been described (Levinson et al., 1978; Greenspan & Pollock, 1980; Nemiroff & Colarusso, 1985). The unifying theme across conceptualizations is linked to a sense of time. The tasks include establishing a career, making decisions regarding marriage and parental roles, addressing issues of midlife change, moving into the latter half of the life cycle with retirement, physical decline, and awareness of death. None of these tasks is achieved in solitude.

THE ROLE OF SOCIAL RELATIONS IN THE RECOVERY FROM ILLNESS

Across all periods of growth, from infancy through old age, the person's capacity to use social relationships for personal satisfaction, support, caring, and stimulation contributes to his or her adjustment and emotional well-being. Many chronically mentally ill persons have significant deficits in their capacity to form and sustain social relationships. Deficiencies in these abilities interfere with individuals' potential to use such resources in their recovery process. For a portion of this population, the deficits can be detected in childhood.

One innovative study illustrates the presence of deficits in children who subsequently were diagnosed as having schizophrenia (Walker & Lewine, 1990). Home movies of children under 8 years of age who later became schizophrenic were compared with those of siblings who remained well. Judges, who were not provided with any criteria by which to identify the preschizophrenic children, were able to make the correct identification beyond that expected from chance. Their observations about the children pointed to less responsiveness, eye contact, and positive affect. They noted poor fine and gross motor coordination. These and other peculiarities may act to estrange children in their interaction with peers and family, which in turn would tend to diminish their self-esteem.

Research assessing premorbid functioning that may contribute to development of a serious psychiatric disorder has focused primarily on children in schizophrenic families. Goldstein (1990) reviewed the research on preonset vulnerability markers. Neurointegrative functions that refer to neuromotor attentional autonomic nervous system reactivity and cognitive processes have all been investigated. Goldstein summarizes the studies as follows:

> Children of schizophrenic parents show a number of early signs and dysfunctions that discriminate them from their peers. Typically, however,

only a subsample of the offspring shows these signs and dysfunctions, and it appears that it is these offspring who are at greater risk for the disorder.

Most signs of neurointegrative and social deficits do not appear to be specific to the offspring of schizophrenics or unique predictors of subsequent schizophrenia. . . .

There is little evidence as yet that these measures of neurointegrative and social deficits can serve as vulnerability markers in children whose parents have not manifested a schizophrenic disorder. (p. 7)

Commenting on these studies, Goldstein observes, "Generally, when high-risk subjects were compared with children of parents with other forms of psychiatric disorder, the differences were less pronounced than when they were compared with children of normal controls" (p. 4). The search for specific predictors of future pathology continues, but the neurodevelopmental processes may act to counter deficits encountered in early childhood.

A person's difficulties interacting socially have a tendency to be self-perpetuating. Children who are different, who are peculiar or clumsy, who are lacking in social skills tend to be ostracized by their playmates. A cycle may be established in which the vulnerable child or adolescent reaches out, only to be rejected or emotionally injured. The result may be withdrawal or aggression that further exaggerates social deficits. These experiences are background for chronically ill persons who may desire more satisfactory social contact, but internally erect barriers against intimacy as an attempt to avoid being emotionally traumatized again.

Helping individuals overcome their deficits in interpersonal functioning has proven difficult. Treatments have been designed to overcome specific observable behavioral deficits. A variety of educational and psychotherapeutic efforts have been devised to address underlying emotional dynamics that interfere with engaging in satisfactory personal relationships. The next section will review several studies that examine patients' experiences of recovery from mental illness and their perception of the role of social relationships in the maintenance of their quality of life.

CLINICAL STUDIES

Erickson et al. (1989) assessed the relationship between improvement and characteristics and involvement in social networks of seriously ill persons. Measures of social network, availability of social resources, and perceived social support were correlated with Axis V (Global Assessment of Functioning) ratings at 18-month follow-up for 46 persons diagnosed with schizophrenia and 49 with affective psychosis experiencing their initial episode of illness. The authors conclude, "In general, correlations between predictor variables and 18-month Axis V ratings provided strong support for the hypothesis that greater involvement with and higher quality of social relationships make for better prognosis in schizophrenia" (p. 1458).

Thornicroft and Breakey (1991) reported that "contact," defined as meeting three times weekly outside of clinic settings with outreach workers for more than 1 year, led to improved social relationships in schizophrenic patients, when compared with those who maintained contact for less than a year. No significant alterations in cognitive functioning, symptoms, or global functioning were found across the study period. Continuing contact with professional helpers appears to have a positive impact on social relations, but may not alter symptoms or overall functioning.

Lehman (1983) used a structured interview that assessed the global well-being of 278 "mentally disabled" residents in licensed board and care homes in Los Angeles County. Two-thirds of the participants were male, 75% were white, and over 50% had never married. Their diagnoses included schizophrenia (63%), alcoholism (11%), organic brain syndrome (9%), personality disorder (9%), and substance abuse (4%). The patients' self-reported senses of global well-being were associated with satisfaction with health and leisure activities, and to a lesser extent, with social relations and finances. Objective measures that correlated with well-being included being satisfied with work, not being a victim of crime, using less health care, and having greater measures of intimate social contacts.[1] Their responses reflect a concern for health and safety, followed by satisfaction with social relationships.

Thase and Howland (1994) reviewed studies assessing psychosocial correlates of depression refractory to pharmacotherapy. Such factors as serious personality pathology, dysfunctional interpersonal attitudes, and long-term marital discord interfered with medication response (Goering et al., 1992) and enhanced the potential for chronicity. Removing barriers to forming successful relationships presumably would enhance treatment response. Clinicians treating severely depressed persons also are prone to unknowingly withdraw, further eroding their patients' supportive network (Bouhuys & Van den Hoofdakker, 1993).

Taken together, these reports provide evidence that social relationships are important in the recovery from mental illness.[2] In the next section, the role of self-help groups in patients' stabilization and recovery from severe mental illness will be explored.

THE SELF-HELP MOVEMENT

The ability of peer relations to assist in the stabilization and recovery from illness is nowhere illustrated as powerfully as in the self help movement. Recovery Inc., begun in the 1930s under the leadership of Abraham A. Low, a psychiatrist, created a structure that was helpful to many mentally ill persons. The success of Alcoholics Anonymous (AA) in assisting many individuals to combat their alcoholism has been a clear indicator of the success of peer support in the "recovering" process.

The growth of self-help organizations in the latter half of the century has been spectacular. Brown (1988) estimated that 12 million people belonged to self-help organizations, a figure that had doubled in the prior 12 years. The rapid increase paralleled the social changes taking place in American culture. The civil rights movement seemed to energize the country and underserved and disenfranchised segments of the population organized to promote change (Katz & Bender, 1976). Self-help groups provided services to "populations" that were neglected or received insufficient attention from establishment caregivers. The National Alliance for the Mentally Ill (NAMI) emerged from a conference organized in the fall of 1979 by a group of families of persons with mental illness in Dane County (Madison), Wisconsin. Nearly 300 people registered, and within the weekend, the energy stimulated by the conference produced the beginnings of a national organization, with an agreed upon name, purpose, and funding mechanism (Howe & Howe, 1987). The subsequent political and educational activities of NAMI have become very important in efforts to destigmatize and change the social environment for patients and families.

Self-help groups espouse a variety of goals and may vary in their commitment to such goals. Katz and Bender (1976) proposed a five-fold topology for self-help groups: (1) groups primarily focused on self-fulfillment or personal growth, (2) groups promoting social advocacy, (3) groups that create alternative patterns for living, (4) "outcast haven" or "rock bottom" groups, and (5) groups of a mixed type. Alternative classifications examined the degree of political and educational activities that attempt to inform the public or change the social norms (e.g., NAMI) and those that are more focused on providing support within the social framework, such as Recovery Inc., GROW Inc., or Emotions Anonymous.

The diversity of goals and organizational structures provides a number of pathways in which disaffected individuals may participate and relieve their suffering. Actively engaging in political action, social reform, educational enterprises, or group meetings may enlarge an individual's social network in a positively reinforcing manner, thereby contributing to the person's well-being. An additional distinction is drawn between "primary" groups for former mental patients and "secondary" groups comprised of parents and relatives of mental patients (Emerick, 1989).

Lieberman (1990) has examined the dynamic properties of support groups that are directed toward personal change. He suggests that the sense of belonging to a homogeneous group, sharing of concerns, cognitive learning linked to new knowledge of the illness process or of coping methods contributes to stabilization and change. Individuals enter into groups often with intense suffering, and their wish for relief combined with the requirement of sharing, decreases their sense of isolation. In the process, participants hear about veteran members' successes, which creates a sense of hope. These are powerful dynamics that enhance the sense of belonging and create a cohesive group that can exert influence on its members. Change has to come from the individual, and externalization of problems is not accepted. Thus the norm characteristic of many groups promoting personal responsibility is more readily accepted.

Cognitive restructuring—new ways of thinking of old problems—is an additional characteristic of self-help groups that contributes to change. Specific suggestions prescribing how to think about anxiety or manage the reemergence of other symptoms become part of the lore of groups that serve to help in times of crises. Availability of members to help others in crises serves as an additional reinforcer of the group's ideology and the individual's growth (Young & Williams, 1988).

Recovery Inc. represents one highly organized, well-structured model that emphasizes cognitive restructuring (Wechsler, 1960). At each weekly meeting, members review portions of Dr. Low's (1950) book, *Mental Health Through Will-Training*, and apply his system in their daily lives. The method includes a number of maxims that are learned to manage stress, for example, (1) the psychoneurotic or postpsychotic symptom is distressing but not dangerous, and (2) tenseness intensifies and sustains the symptom and thus should be avoided.

Following reading or listening to tapes, members describe recent experiences in which they have applied the method. Peer leaders are selected from among members and are trained by more senior leaders and an official guidebook.

Galenter (1988) surveyed leaders and individuals who had been members of Recovery Inc. for periods of 6 to 24 months. He found that individuals reported less distress after joining. The leaders, who were long-term members, used less psychotropic medications and psychotherapy than newer members. Gallenter concluded that well-structured peer-led groups, which utilized cognitive materials, could be of value as an adjunct to psychiatric treatment.

Concerns that some persons may be harmed by the more zealous groups have been raised. Such groups have a very strong ideology and tend to be extremely stressful for those who do not adhere to their standards and become alienated from the group (Galenter, 1990). Anecdotal stories suggest that groups have the potential to be harmful, particularly in circumstances in which norms have been violated. Individuals may then be stressed by conflicting wishes to belong and to maintain their own standards that violate the group norm. The extent of such negative effects is uncertain.

Overall, the popularity and the growth of the self-help movement is testimony to suffering individuals' search for ways to relieve their distress and, either as a primary or secondary benefit, make connections with others. The measures of effectiveness are not well documented, but the overwhelming thrust of personal testimonials and the small amount of research suggest that the movement serves an important personal and societal need. There appears to be increasing acceptance by conventional clinicians of support groups as an adjunct to treatment.

Within the traditional psychotherapeutic community, a series of strategies have emerged that are designed to assist patients in overcoming their social isolation and improving relationships. The following sections selectively review family therapy and expressed emotion and social skills training, which are treatment strategies addressing deficits in patients' interpersonal functioning.

FAMILY THERAPY AND EXPRESSED EMOTION

Not surprisingly, clinicians began to examine the family system as the prototype for disturbed social relations. If relationships were disturbed in the family, then family treatment might alter the pathology and free the patient to interact more satisfactorily. Steinglass (1987) traced the shifting focus in family therapy for schizophrenia. He observes that early contributors to these studies (e.g., Bateson, Lidz, Fleck, Wynne, and Singer) emphasized specific intrafamilial communicational distortions that essentially pointed the finger at the family as the causative agent for the illness—the "schizophrenogenic mother." Family treatment within this theoretical framework was often very confrontational and was designed to change the family pathology. In essence, the family, particularly the mother, was blamed for the schizophrenic person's illness.

The initial enthusiasm for this treatment approach diminished as disturbed communicational patterns were not found to be specific to these families. Moreover, research findings from twin and adoption studies altered the weight of evidence to a major biological–genetic basis for this illness.

Studies of the family influence on the *course* rather than the etiology of schizophrenia have replaced the earlier models. The construct of expressed emotion followed from the observations of Brown et al. (1958) that chronic schizophrenic men who lived with wives or parents were more likely to relapse than those who lived independently or with other relatives. Brown et al. (1962), from interviews with patients and family members, initially correlated five factors with relapse: (1) emotion of any valence directed toward the patient, (2) hostility directed toward the patient, (3) dominant behavior toward the patient, (4) emotion expressed by the patient toward relatives, and (5) hostility expressed by the patient toward relatives. These factors were subsequently modified and became the basis of an interview schedule (the Camberwell Interview). Tabulation of the ratings from the interview produced scores that were dichotomized into high and low expressed emotion.[3]

A series of studies were consistent in replicating Brown's initial findings that patients living in low-expressed-emotion families were not likely to decompensate in the first 9–12 months posthospitalization (Falloon et al., 1982; Leff et al., 1982; Leff, Kuipers, Berkowitz, & Sturgeon, 1985; Hogarty et al., 1986).

Schizophrenic patients' premorbid personality characteristics of social inactivity and withdrawal were found to be associated with high expressed emotion (Kuipers, 1979; Runions & Prudo, 1983). High expressed emotion in the family was not associated with the patients' acute symptoms but instead was correlated with negative symptoms.

Treatment strategies were developed that shifted away from blaming families toward educational efforts in which the biological stress model of illness was highlighted. Families were provided information about the nature and course of the illness, and they were taught methods of stress reduction designed to decrease expressed emotion. Interventions utilizing a psychoeducational model demonstrated significant reduction in relapse rates for patients who were also receiving medication in the 9- to 12-month posthospital follow-up period, when compared with subjects not receiving the educational intervention. "Relapse" was carefully defined as reappearance of major symptoms or the necessity for hospitalization (Falloon et al., 1982; Leff et al., 1982, 1985; Hogarty et al., 1986; Kottgen et al., 1984). A report of 2-year outcome showed that family therapy continued to forestall relapse (Hogarty et al., 1991). An additional element that contributed to the protection of patients from relapse was the decrease in family contact time to less than 30 hours weekly.

Critiques of expressed emotion research point out that the authors oversampled schizophrenic patients who were young, unmarried males who resided in parental households. In a pilot study of residential care operators, levels of expressed emotion were found to be less than in a report from a comparable geographic area for families of origin. Positive correlations were found between levels of pathology of schizophrenic and schizoaffective patients and levels of expressed emotion for those living in a residential setting at least 6 months (Snyder et al., 1994). An exception to the generally positive studies is the finding that young women, who are in low-expressed-emotion environments and are separated and/or divorced, experience recurrent exacerbations of their psychotic illness (Hogarty et al., 1990).

Additional studies have examined the impact of expressed emotion on the course of depression (Vaughn & Leff, 1976; Hooley et al., 1986). Depressed patients tend to relapse at considerably lower scores of expressed emotion than do schizophrenic patients. An important difference between the schizophrenic and depressed groups is the much greater proportion of depressive patients living with spouses. Hooley et al. (1986) proposed that the "sensitivity" in depressed patients may be linked to a greater threat of separation or loss in the marital relationship than exists in schizophrenic persons' families.

In a summary of the literature on expressed emotion, Koenigsberg and Handley (1986) stated: "Expressed emotion is a concept legitimized by its predictive validity; its meaning and construct validity remain to be established" (p. 1367)[4] Despite those theoretical limitations, the vulnerability of seriously mentally ill patients to intense affect stimulation, particularly feelings and expression of anger, and of too great a demand for involvement, has implications for the conduct of group psychotherapy in which an emphasis is placed on recognition and expression of anger and regular and prompt attendance.

SOCIAL SKILLS TRAINING

In view of the disability of chronically mentally ill persons, it is not surprising to see efforts to modify and improve their social skills deficits through behavioral approaches. Brady (1984) reviewed the basic concepts of social skills, which he suggested was a general term that encompassed under- and overassertiveness, and verbal and nonverbal expressiveness. Social skills may be categorized as affectional and instrumental. Individuals exhibiting affectional deficits are described as awkward when they attempt to be friendly to strangers and acquaintances. Individuals exhibiting instrumental deficits have difficulties in community living, including use of transportation, health resources, and social services. Two models of training have developed: motor skills and social functioning (Bellack et al., 1989). The motor skills model assumes that effective social functioning is a result of smooth integration of a set of specific behavioral elements, including verbal responses, paralinguistic (i.e., voice, tone, and volume) and nonverbal features. The social functioning, "problem-solving" model focuses on the patient's inability to process social inputs (recognition of partner's emotions) and to engage in effective problem solving.

Behavioral training of social skills for schizophrenic patients has had limited success. Skills taught in the laboratory or in training settings are not readily generalized to everyday living situations (Liberman et al., 1986; Hogarty et al., 1991).

Interest has shifted to gaining understanding of significant deficits in a wide range of cognitive processes in schizophrenic individuals. These include memory, attention, reasoning ability, and language usage (Neuchterlein & Dawson, 1984; Braff & Geyer, 1990). Faulty cognitive processing is assumed to be a major contributor to social skills deficits. One assumption is that many of the successful therapies utilized in treating brain-injured persons can be employed with schizophrenic patients (Spring & Ravdin, 1992). However, this assumption is controversial (Bellack, 1992).

Continuing efforts at overcoming cognitive and associated social skills deficits with behavioral training suffer from lack of an overarching model. The report of Hogarty et al., (1991) provides some evidence that continued reinforcement is necessary to sustain gains, and interruption of contact with the clinician results in loss of previously attained gains. Leff believes that schizophrenia is associated with a continuing vulnerability for the patient, and, therefore, he does not terminate treatment (personal communication, 1992).

Deficits in social skills frequently emerge in groups with the chronically mentally ill. Clinicians may opt to have members practice certain assertive skills, such as asking for directions or speaking up to have needs satisfied, or they may address patients' lack of eye contact. Patients may temporarily respond to the specific recommendation, but they may have difficulty sustaining their gains or generalizing them. Despite these limitations, a piece of new learning in the group may have a beneficial effect on in-group processes such as cohesion.

SUMMARY

In this chapter, the functions of interpersonal relationships in human development have been briefly reviewed as a background for examining the place of social interaction in recovery from chronic mental illness. Social relationships have an impact on the adult individual's capacity to tolerate stress and to recover from mental illness. The patient's capacity to develop and sustain useful networks, inside and outside the family, reflects an individual's personal development and the availability and capacities of those in the network.

The meteoric increase in support groups, with broad testimonial approval, is an indicator of the social needs of chronically mentally ill individuals. The nature of the support movement, which limits contact with professionals, may have interfered with adequate research examining the benefits of this broad movement. Nevertheless, it appears that clinicians treating this population are more willing to encourage patients to seek additional help through joining a support group. Indeed, many substance abuse programs include support groups as an intrinsic element in their rehabilitation strategies.

Two major treatment models—expressed emotion and social skills training—have emerged in an effort to modify the course of major illness. The research in expressed emotion has shown that this treatment strategy will modify relapse rates in schizophrenic and depressed individuals. The sustained benefit of social skills training is insufficiently documented, and newer approaches to understanding the cognitive basis for these deficits are underway.

It would be premature to suggest more than the most tentative of conclusions, but the work with expressed emotion suggests that clinicians may need to pay particular attention to the chronically ill patient's affect tolerance and integration. Excessive affect stimulation interferes with cognitive functioning and may intrude on learning or sustaining social skills.

With the increasing emphasis on pharmacotherapy as the major therapeutic agent in the treatment of chronic illness, this review demonstrates that there is a substantial body of knowledge supporting the beneficial place of social relationships and treatment strategies aimed at improving these relationships in the outcome of chronic illness. The words of an anonymous recovering patient (1986) succinctly summarize the needs of a chronically ill individual:

> I have learned that some of the basic elements of my illness may have been present since early childhood, in which case the way I related to my family and early acquaintances must have been affected and probably influenced the way other people related to me, even on an unconscious level. If this is true, the confusion I felt about myself was compounded by what seemed irrational or conflicting actions directed toward me. A child destined to become schizophrenic must deal not only with the seeds of the illness within himself but also with the attitudes of others toward his "idiosyncrasies," whether these feelings are voiced openly or subtly manifested in everyday life. Even if medication can free the schizophrenic patient from some of his torment, the scars of emotional confusion remain, felt perhaps more deeply by a greater sensitivity and vulnerability. . . .
>
> Psychotherapy, in combination with drug therapy, supportive emotional day treatment, and a weekly group therapy session, has worked for me. Most of my program supports psychotherapy, which I consider the center of my treatment. . . . (pp. 68–69)

FIVE

GROUP DYNAMICS AND DEVELOPMENT

The discipline (a few shared values) provides the framework. It gives people confidence (to experiment, for instance) stemming from stable expectations about what really counts.

—PETERS & WATERMAN (1982, p. 322)

undamental to the process of helping individuals benefit from their psychotherapeutic encounters is an understanding of the factors that contribute to or inhibit change. As described by Peters and Waterman, structures exist in successful companies that enable individuals to experiment and try new ideas within a context that they understand encourages rather than punishes experimentation and innovation. These are some of the dynamics of successful companies. Group dynamics are the assumed forces that mobilize change. In this chapter, I will examine the elements that can be assigned primarily to the forces within the group field that impact on the individual. This focus is by its very nature arbitrary, because group dynamics are reverberating processes that impact on and change the individual, who in turn, impacts on the group. This cycle optimally leads to expanding health.

GROUP DYNAMICS

The study of group dynamics has been confused by the incomplete differentiation of the processes contributed from two separate traditions:

(1) that of the analytic clinician focusing on the individual, and (2) that of the sociologist studying the properties of the group (Durkin, 1957). Slavson (1957), writing within the analytic tradition, questioned the presence of group dynamics in therapy groups. He was attempting to illustrate that the individual and group dynamic perspectives were not compatible in the conduct of a psychotherapy group. In the extensive clinical example, Slavson focused exclusively on the personal history of each of the women in the group in order to understand the meaning of their interaction with him, the leader and sole male present. A reader of the vignette who maintains a systems focus on the interaction will readily observe the members' intense competition for the leader's attention and admiration, a dynamic ignored by Slavson. The paper actually accomplished the opposite of the author's intent to illustrate the superordinate position of individual dynamics. Instead, it served to broaden many clinicians' understanding of the relationship between individual and group dynamics.

Group dynamics encompass the view of the group as a social field in which elements of leadership, status, roles, structure, climate, standards, pressure, and communication are in interaction (Durkin, 1957). The following discussion, will focus on the central elements of leadership, culture, and roles.

Leadership

One salient model for the dynamic function of the group leader was conceptualized by Freud (1921) as a process in which members of a group idealized the leader and identified with one another. The theoretical basis for this formulation was derived from Freud's examination of the Oedipus conflict and the childhood relationship to a father figure. Later theoreticians (Glatzer, 1965; Scheidlinger, 1974) focused on preoedipal dynamics, in which the leader was ambivalently experienced in the transference as a maternal object who was to provide basic elements of safety and care, or who was potentially destructively engulfing.

The object relations tradition evolved from the work of Melanie Klein and, in particular, in the theorizing of Wilfred Bion (1961). Bion focused on omnipresent basic assumption life that intrudes upon the goal-oriented, reality functioning of a group, in which members, operating in concert, respond *as if* they are meeting to gratify emotional needs. Bion posited three basic assumptions, those of dependency, fight–flight, and pairing. Basic assumption dynamics have been understood as responses to the object relation needs revolving around a "leader." Group leadership encompasses the therapist as a real person (work group) and as a transference (basic assumption, mythical) figure, or it may be distributed among attributes of members or assigned to the group as a whole (e.g., a fight group).

In addition, Bion speculated that each person possessed an innate tendency (valence) to act on one of the basic assumptions. This latter theoretical notion, although not substantiated, has been utilized by clinicians to explain human beings' attraction to groups.

A significant element in the therapist's work is his or her serving as a container for group emotions. Feelings are projected into the clinician, who may understand and "metabolize" them. The affects experienced by the therapist may be interpreted to the members in order for them to gain self-understanding.

The individual dynamic perspective examines the ambivalent responses to the group therapist. The leader represents a source of love, protection, and needs satisfaction, but also represents control, power, and destruction. The potential for the leader to be a focus for a host of projections becomes clear in this context.

From the sociological perspective, the leader has the task of establishing goals and structure. The externally directed functions include defining boundaries, membership, group size, time, and duration of sessions. Defining the composition, recruiting members, and preparing them for entry significantly impact upon the functioning of the group. Defining the size and composition of the membership and duration of the meeting impact upon how much time is available for each individual and consequently affects the intermember relationships. For example, a group that has one or two widely deviant members (across a broad continuum of dimensions) will most likely develop differently from a group composed more homogeneously.

Leaders manage internal dynamics that encompass setting of initial group standards, norms, and values. Whether this is accomplished by spelling out these expectations verbally or in writing, or by utilizing the authority of the leadership role to reinforce desired behaviors in the evolving process, the leader's position is powerful, but not the only element, in achieving the desired standards. The group contract, which is the initial agreement between members and the clinician, is an overt manifestation of the therapist's management activities. Members' initial and continuing expectations of the group and the leader and their ability to tolerate and work with anxiety and conflict act to modify the initial agreements and can be viewed as the processes in which norms and values are altered.

The leader must have the resources necessary to assist the members in working toward their goals. These resources are in part based on the external world, such as the availability of referrals to group, and in part on their own personal characteristics and values that influence the focus of their attention.

Newton (1973) has proposed a linkage between individual and sociological based dynamics. The external boundarying functions, he suggests, are similar to the traditional paternal tasks external to the family, such as providing the resources in which the family can function. In groups, these functions would include recruiting and screening members, negotiating for space, administrative support, and so on. The internal boundary management is similar to maternal functions in which the mother provides nurturing, expectations of development, and conflict resolution within the family bounds. These are aspects of the leadership role that evoke both maternal and paternal transferences to the therapist.

Culture

The culture of the group is a product of the leader's expectations, members' interactions, and their fantasies about the group as a whole. In a therapy group, the culture is influenced to a significant degree by the members' capacity to tolerate anxiety, willingness to take risks, and their capacity for change. The theoretical concepts of the group focal conflict (Whitaker & Lieberman, 1964) are illustrative of culture formation. In this model, members interact until some common wish (which may not be conscious) is stimulated. In most situations, this wish is met with a fantasied negative reaction and, as a result, a compromise formation (a solution) emerges that will partially gratify the wish and not evoke too much anxiety. The flexibility of solutions that enables progress toward group goals (enabling solutions) or inhibits progress (restrictive solutions) represents the group climate and culture. A similar model based on the triad of impulse, counterimpulse, and solution is evident in the object relations theory of Ezriel (1973).

Embedded in the concept of group culture is that of norms. Group norms are not a result of conscious decisions in relation to what is or is not acceptable, but they are a product of group interaction. For example, the therapist may attempt to establish a norm that members directly express feelings about their in-group interactions. Members' efforts to comply (out of a wish to please the therapist) may evoke unmanageable anxiety in one or several members, and as a consequence, the group "decides" that it will remain friendly, nonconfrontative, and discuss external topics. From a group-focal-conflict perspective, these actions would represent restrictive solutions.

Norms are established about all aspects of the group life and serve to contain anxiety. Groups may develop prohibitions against too intense expressions of intimacy. Flirtation or sexual competition may be ignored, or "offending" members may be told directly that such feelings are not acceptable in the group. Continued violation of a norm may be met with sanctions, not infrequently in the form of ostracism or scapegoating.

The broader social culture contributes to what members will freely discuss. For instance, money in the American culture often represents power, status, and achievement. In groups composed of successful individuals, the specific details of a person's wealth and expenditures are rarely discussed. It would seem quite gauche, too, for a member to ask another how much was spent on a vacation or for a spouse's birthday gift. In contrast, working with chronically mentally ill patients, who have far fewer monetary resources, the topic of money often is addressed directly as members share their experiences purchasing clothing and food, or with agencies providing entitlement funds. The group cultures, as differentiated by social class, evolve differently.

A group that develops a culture that is attractive to its members and can satisfy members' emotional needs as well as their personal goals becomes cohesive. The interpersonal field in the context of cohesion has much greater influence on members' behavior. Yalom (1985) states, "Group cohesiveness is not *per se* a therapeutic factor but is instead a necessary precondition for effective therapy" (p. 50). An alternative viewpoint is put forth in the theories of self psychology. A group culture in which members would have their needs empathically understood may restabilize a disorganizing self, and the person may then proceed to continue previously blocked development (Stone, 1992). This framework provides an explanation for so-called transference cures and some premature terminations.

Roles

Roles can be considered a function of the group, in which the group's need and an individual's personality characteristics interact. MacKenzie (1990) suggests that four roles derived from the sociological literature are identifiable in therapy groups: sociable, structural, divergent, and cautionary. These roles may be filled by a particular individual with a propensity to behave in the necessary fashion, or they may be filled by several members who provide the function. A member may be "sucked into" a role to fulfill a group need and, as a consequence, experience considerable dysphoria (Redl, 1942)

The sociable role essentially is one that monitors the intensity of the interpersonal relationships and attempts to build positive relations. The role includes the host or hostess who greets the newcomers, or it may be the soother who breaks tension with a joke or a shift of topic. The group's need for this function varies with the members' ability to tolerate anxiety and to work together on difficult issues, and therefore, it may be prominent at one point in the life of the group and not in another.

The sociable role, as with any other function, may become exaggerated out of needs of the group and from that perspective inhibit change as the members become stuck being pleasant to one another. An individual who habitually fills this role then may become an easy target to be scapegoated, as will be discussed in the deviant role.

The structural role is similar to that of the task leader. The role includes a cognitive component that emphasizes understanding of where the group is headed, the tasks that are being addressed, and what needs to be accomplished. In a sophisticated group, this role may be filled by the member who tries to understand the process preceding an affective outburst. In a newly forming group, this role may fall to those who share their experiences or asks others to share theirs. It may be the person who examines feelings in relation to boundary violations, such as a member's lateness that has been ignored. It might include the person who raises questions about the discussion being focused on outside events rather than group interaction, or the individual who translates the discussion as a metaphor for experiences in the group. Many of these functions initially are carried out by the therapist, but members may enter the group with certain skills in this direction or they may acquire them as part of their learning in the treatment process.

The divergent role most often is associated with the scapegoat. This role can be overt or subtle. The scapegoat is traditionally seen as the person who carries unacceptable affects and is ostracized into the "wilderness." The members disavow feelings as unacceptable and place them in the designated recipient. A member may express too much hostility at a given point, or a confrontation may be seen as too harsh, and although others may have similar feelings (often not consciously recognized), they isolate them in the offending person. Similarly, expressions of erotic love (whether heterosexual or homosexual) can produce considerable dysphoria and lead to scapegoating. Divergence can be expressed against any of the emerging group norms. Absences without notification, tardiness, gossiping, and nonpayment of fees are examples of such behaviors. The role usually stirs considerable affect and promotes interaction. This can serve very powerful and productive forces, but if the affective stimulation is greater than can be managed, then there is potential for the member to be sacrificed.

The fourth role is that of the cautionary member. Generally, this is the member who does not reveal very much. These individuals may sit quietly or intellectualize their responses, thereby keeping themselves at some distance from the others. All people have secrets and aspects of themselves that they are anxious about exposing, and the cautionary member provides the personification of those elements. The cautious member also contains for the group a belief that self-disclosure is dangerous and members can be extremely hurtful toward one another. The overlap between the cautionary and divergent roles is considerable.

Not all behavior fulfills social roles. An individual's unique characteristics may be fundamentally irrelevant to the group. Initially, the individual may be considered to be in the divergent role and fulfill a group function. For instance, a person who needs to be the center of attention and monopolizes the group may protect the others from revealing themselves or may become a focus of all of the hostility in the group and protect the members from other intermember conflict. In the monopolizer's absence, the group may chat about trivial topics or they may be very nice to one another. Such behaviors would tend to confirm the presence of a group role. If this role were solely that of the particular individual and not salient to the others, considerable therapeutic movement might take place in his or her absence. In that scenario, the individual role would be most pronounced.

The concepts of leadership, norms, culture, and roles are applicable to all groups. Appreciation of the dynamic elements that impact on the members of a therapy group broadens the clinicians understanding of patterns of members' interaction.

GROUP DEVELOPMENT

It should come as no surprise that the nature of relationships changes among individuals in the course of time. What is somewhat surprising is that there is a broad, orderly sequence to those changes that is subsumed under the concept of group development. The developmental stages can be characterized by members trying to accomplish different tasks and simultaneously meet their emotional needs. In a psychotherapy group, there is considerable overlap between the goals of improved emotional functioning and attention to the individual's emotional needs. Despite the potential confusion, it is useful for the clinician to separate these two aspects of group interactions (Bennis & Shepard, 1956; Tuckman, 1965).

Beginning Phase

The task of persons entering a psychotherapy group is determining how they can achieve their goals through their participation. There are few rules, and even those people who have had prior group experiences still face the task of joining with a number of strangers where the norms and culture are not established. One aspect of prior experiences makes sense—to look for direction and signposts from the designated leader, the therapist. If the therapist's responses do not fulfill members' expectations, they might look for others who have had experiences in therapy groups as a next step. Many patients in groups for the chronically mentally ill have been hospitalized and might fall back on their experience with groups in the hospital. Individuals spontaneously draw on previous experiences to help orient themselves. The human tendency to repeat strategies that were effective in uncharted situations is familiar to all. What works in one place or time, however, may not work in another.

A patient might share a problem, hoping to obtain a solution. Others frequently will give advice in an effort to be helpful. Generally, such advice is of minimal value, because the person offering up a problem is cautious about what he or she reveals and probably has previously received similar advice. Nevertheless, members' suggestions may be responded to eagerly as a bit of evidence that participating in the group can be useful. Contrariwise, suggestions may be taken in and then rejected as evidence that only the therapist can provide anything useful.

Concomitant with these interactions, members are working to determine the rules of behavior. What can we discuss? What should we avoid? How should I participate? The evolution of these rules establishes group norms and culture. The boundaries of the task also are explored. Can I come late? How often can I miss? What happens when I hug someone in the group? How about hugging outside the session?

The emotional needs of the members in this phase are very much center stage. A person's emotional requirements for safety are stimulated when the nature of the task is unclear. Other members are strangers, and they represent both an opportunity and a threat, but the therapist at least is a somewhat known quantity, assuming that appropriate screening and preparatory interviews have taken place. The pregroup interviews spent preparing a new member represents a beginning relationship and adds to the member's dependency upon the therapist.

Stranger anxiety, which is present in everyone in varying degrees, is compounded when the task is to greet a group of individuals and reveal one's problems, including guilty and shameful secrets. Some articulate individuals are able to describe a deep-seated fear of being sucked up into an unknown morass; they fear they will lose themselves and cease to exist; their individual boundaries are threatened with dissolution. Successful efforts from the past to overcome this anxiety are called into play. Patients try to safely engage others by asking socially safe questions. Where do you live? What is your work? Are you married? They look for similarities that will decrease the anxiety, or they withdraw and adopt a cautionary role. Questions of a person's capacities for basic trust, risk taking, and acting on feelings are all brought into focus in this initial stage.

As in all groups, those composed of chronically mentally ill individuals exhibit opening stage dynamics that are intertwined with patients' personal developmental level. Patients try to determine if the group is trustworthy, and they carefully explore whether they will be emotionally traumatized in the current situation as they have been in the past. Members, not infrequently, go through extended periods of withdrawal or regression to somatization or even to psychotic thinking in this stage. Fears of losing one's self or that personal boundaries are fragile and will not withstand more than superficial contact are some of the elements that represent ego weakness and are the source of a patient's caution. If members do interact spontaneously, their remarks are usually directed to the therapist in the form of a question. Cooper (1978) describes the earliest entry phase for chronically ill persons as a pregroup stage in which only the patient and the therapist seem to exist. The therapist must be active in reinforcing tentative efforts by members to contact peers in assisting movement through the pregroup phase.

When members in this phase begin to respond to peers, their behavior is similar to that of children playing in a sandbox. They all are playing, but they are not interacting. The comments of one member may evoke associations to similar experiences in others. Those associations are not directly linked to the initiator of the discussion. The conversation flows as if each person is metaphorically building his or her own castle in the sand. The therapist (mother) may be looked to for approval, but only furtive glances are exchanged with the others in the sandbox. Thus, the therapist in this stage has the central role and others may listen to what is taking place, but they generally will not enter into the interaction.

Subgrouping is a common phenomenon in the entry phase. Frequently, patients come to the group via public transportation, and they soon make arrangements to meet and come together, or conversely, they ride home together. Sometimes those with cars will offer others rides. These are nascent ways of forming some ties among members. Ordinarily, these dyads or triads are mentioned in the group without evoking overt jealousy, which is in keeping with members' reluctance (or fear) to tackle intragroup affects. Members may spontaneously exchange full names and phone numbers, which would be unusual for members of higher functioning groups. Generally this is a positive step, but on occasion a person who feels excluded may terminate from the group.

Eventually, if the therapist proves to be sufficiently reliable and attempts to understand the emotional needs of the members, they will begin to reach out and interact more directly with one another and move toward the second developmental stage.

Because of the fragility of many patients, passage into the second stage may be uneven, and patients easily return to earlier modes of functioning. It would be a mistake for the therapist to hurry patients to complete this phase. It is the building block for future personal and group development.

Patients require sufficient time to solidify basic trust and a sense of safety with the therapist as well as participate in nontraumatic experiences with peers before they will risk moving to the next stage.

The Interactive Phase

Developmental models with higher functioning individuals conceptualize a second developmental stage as one of rebellion and striving for autonomy (Bennis & Shepard, 1956; Rutan & Stone, 1993). Members have dealt with their dependency wishes focused on the therapist, and they have established norms of behavior that are often experienced as rigid. A basic sense of trust in the therapist and themselves has developed, enabling members to feel a degree of confidence in their own resources. They are in an emotional position to overthrow their therapist.

Members rid themselves of "dependency" upon the leader and clash over peer power. An aura of rebelliousness is woven into the fabric of the sessions. Whose rules are going to be followed? How much independence may I have and remain a member? The rebellions shift from those directed to the leader, and in their place, struggles arise against the perception of inflexibility of group norms and values. Successful negotiation of this phase leads to greater flexibility of group norms, a greater tolerance for affect, and some resolution of member–leadership struggles.

This image of group development does not coincide with what is observed in groups of the chronically mentally ill. The therapist remains important to the members, who seem to require reassurance that they will not be prematurely emotionally abandoned. There is greater member-to-member interaction, with genuine sharing of experiences, advice giving, and relevant associations to emotional stimuli. There is a degree of continuity, and members may inquire about significant events in one another's lives that were mentioned in previous sessions: for example, "How is your mother after her surgery?" "Were you able to meet with your social worker and fix the spindown?"[1] Such inquiries signal a growing level of interest in others' personal lives.

Negative feelings about the treatment or the therapist are generally suppressed or expressed in a displacement, and overt evidence of rebellion is generally limited, often emerging through absences, lateness, or other forms of avoidance. Direct expression of frustration or anger at the therapist is unusual. When it is expressed, generally, others will either overtly ignore the comment or disagree. Members do not experience or withhold angry or rageful feelings, in part because of their uncertainty of being able to maintain their own psychic integrity. More commonly, individuals will indicate that they fear retaliation.

Disappointments are communicated more directly but also may be presented in a displacement or through metaphor. Feelings of belonging to a group may reawaken emotional aspects of a person's family of origin. Sometimes members' direct associations link their families with the group.

> *Example*: In one group, Paula, diagnosed with schizophrenia, described her sister's death and their long-standing enmity. She did not go to the funeral, fearing she would get upset. Randy, also suffering from schizophrenia, promptly associated that it was very important for families to stick together and began irritably challenging Paula for her avoidant behavior. In this context, Randy was communicating that he wanted the "family/group" to behave in ways he deemed proper. He seemed unable to listen to a range of experiences and feelings.

> *Example*: A second illustration comes from a group solidly into the second phase that was regularly videotaped. An initial stress was the departure of the regular camera operator, followed within a brief period by the departure of the resident cotherapist. There were no immediate replacements for either person. The group continued under the single leadership of a senior staff member who routinely turned on the video camera, which was left running in a fixed position during the meeting. At the beginning of one session shortly after the cotherapist's departure, one of the members inquired if someone had been found to run the camera. The question was answered in the negative. Part way into the session, the theme of abandonment and unavailable parents emerged. The therapist then connected this theme with the initial question regarding the videotaping and wondered if the members were concerned about the loss of staff and the lack of replacements. The responses were muted, but the underlying fears were that the therapist would leave (he had been away a year previously for an extended period) and that no replacement would be available. Even though this concern was directly addressed by the therapist, the members talked about their feelings that others were not interested in them, and that people would not sit next to them on the bus, or somehow could tell they were mentally ill and avoided them. The topic was fruitful, but direct expression of disappointment, frustration, or anger with the therapist was not forthcoming.

In this context, the focus of patients' sense of control remains external. They have only a nascent sense that they have personal control over their lives. In many ways, this is an accurate assessment, because most receive monies from public funds or they may have a payee who controls their funds. There are significant sectors of their lives in which they do have the potential for control, and there are some attempts to more actively engage in effective problem solving. These dynamics are reflected in continuing, but attenuated, reliance on the therapist.

Movement toward Integration and Autonomy

In this phase, there is evidence of more consistent recognition of individual differences. Stereotypes of people are diminished, and members show an appreciation for more complex feeling states in others. There is less splitting into all good and all bad, and a concomitant recognition that individuals may harbor conflicted feelings.

Sexual feelings are intermittently expressed, sometimes in an adolescent, shy, or teasing manner. The feelings often seem precariously balanced as expressions both of dependency needs from earlier developmental stages and of more mature affection.

In general, affects are better tolerated than in early developmental phases. Most notable are angry affects. Not uncommonly, seriously mentally ill patients will present with provocative, opinionated, or angry behavior. In earlier developmental phases, members back off; they change the topic, try to calm the individual, or they may actually leave the session prematurely. In the more advanced phases, having experienced the therapist's ability to work with such persons, there is greater affect tolerance. Less commonly, patients who have had significant inhibitions in expression of angry affects may begin to test the atmosphere with jokes.

> *Example*: In one group a man with a diagnosis of schizoaffective disorder started the session by telling a rather benign psychiatrist joke; this was followed by a woman, diagnosed with schizophrenia, telling a joke about cannibalism, and the first patient asked, "What do they find in the showers of cannibals? Head and shoulders." A third patient, also diagnosed with schizophrenia, then inquired about the fate of a man who had chopped his wife's head off and had been sent to a psychiatric hospital rather than prison.

The patient's freedom to address expressions of hostility and violence in this fashion represents considerable group development in which feelings expressed in this form can be tolerated. The initial, rather benign psychiatrist joke seemed to have been a test of the therapist.

Groups composed primarily of schizophrenic patients may only reach this phase after many years of work. Those composed of more heterogeneous diagnoses can show genuine affection, concern, and caring. Members share information about themselves, and they relate vignettes of success with authority figures.

> *Example*: One elderly woman with dysthymia, diabetes, arthritis, and obesity described how she had experimented taking Tylenol as a supplement to her prescribed nonsteroidal medications for arthritic pain. She experienced considerable relief. She told her internist of her

success, and almost beamed as she described his positive response to her "experiment," and his suggesting that she continue to use this regimen for relief of her pain. The communication within the group was that the therapist also would listen and that he would encourage experimentation.

These are not consistently achieved interactions, and seriously mentally ill patients are vulnerable to actual or anticipated injury that results in return to early modes of functioning. What emerges, however, over extended periods are patients' latent capacities to manage the stresses associated with their illness. They are faced with the disability linked to being mentally ill, and with the general negative social response to mental illness. Patients present with pride their ability to effectively respond to adversity in both sectors of their lives.

Termination

The termination phase of groups for the chronically mentally ill is characterized primarily as a treatment interruption. Seldom are there opportunities for a patient to genuinely say good-bye to the group, because patients seem to have difficult times resolving issues of separation and loss.

Because of the chronicity of illness, many patients may require treatment for the remainder of their lives. Nevertheless, they may terminate from the group, and if continuing medication is necessary, other arrangements may be made to ensure its provision. Such terminations generally occur when patients have been stabilized for lengthy periods, may be attending sessions on a regular but infrequent basis, and have gained sufficient experience with their illness that they can recognize early signs of decompensation. They can be encouraged to return to the group under such circumstances. The clinician should have sufficient alliance with the treatment system that access is kept as simple as possible. Returning individuals should be able to reenter the group with minimal red tape. In this fashion, the therapist conveys a message that the group is available to all according to their needs.

It is not unusual for patients to find work and be unable to return to the group, or return for only one meeting. Yet, almost all clinicians have treated individuals who, with the best hopes, obtain employment and are unable to sustain themselves under the stress of the task. Reassurance that the group is available can have paradoxical meanings. Patients may interpret the therapist's comment as lack of confidence, coinciding with the person's own anxieties, or experience the comment as continuing interest in event of trouble.

A variation on this scenario is created when a patient leaves the community or moves to another portion of the community and is no longer eligible for services in a particular mental health center. This sometimes is planned and sometimes occurs abruptly as a consequence of the patient's illness. Failure to pay rent, or failure to protect property (because of violence or not maintaining sanitary conditions) can lead to a member's forced change of residence and abrupt departure from the group.

The remaining members have an opportunity to address their feelings about loss, and they often are able to associate to losses of their own, particularly loss of parents or siblings. The termination process is influenced by the nature of the departing patient's tenure and quality of interaction in the group. On occasion, a quiet member will abruptly depart, and in the discussion, a great deal of information about the person will be revealed based on previously hidden outside contacts among the members.

Another aspect of terminations in groups for the seriously mentally ill is linked to patients' deaths. Suicide within this population is not rare, and many groups suffer from the loss of a member in this manner (Westermeyer et al., 1991). This is almost invariably disruptive, with increased concerns about recrudescence of mental illness among the remaining members. Many may feel guilt over not having foreseen the suicide. Because there is frequent contact among members between sessions, the guilt is compounded by one or more members having spoken with the deceased patient between sessions or having heard direct suicidal remarks in one of their extragroup contacts. Feelings that they should have notified the therapist or others are prominent in such circumstances. Although it is not always clear, patients may die in accidents that are suggestive of suicidal intent.

Death from medical illness is much more common in these groups than in the general population. Difficulties in obtaining or utilizing available medical care contribute to increased mortality in this population. Patients with chronic medical illness such as cardiovascular disease and diabetes seem to be present in many groups. Those patients' bouts with medical hospitalization frequently lead to discussions about death of parents and fears regarding their own physical well-being.

Thus, members of groups of the seriously mentally ill frequently have experience with terminations and losses. However the issue of a member's termination is often unaddressed or severely attenuated.

SUMMARY

Clinicians' knowledge of dynamic properties of groups adds a dimension to their understanding of the interaction unfolding in the therapeutic process. Leadership functions have a major impact on group formation, but concepts of group norms, culture, and role enable therapists to conceptualize the in-group transactions at a group level, in addition to the more traditional intrapsychic and interpersonal dimensions derived from dyadic work.

Group development differs in several respects from that observed in groups composed of higher functioning individuals. The therapist retains a more central role over the life of the group. Affect tolerance is more limited, but gains in this sector can be regularly observed. Terminations frequently are unplanned and often minimally addressed or altogether avoided by the departing member. Suicide and death from medical causes are more common in these groups and present an additional termination situation.

SIX

INITIATING
A GROUP PROGRAM

*Since each part of any enterprise has its own primary task
and thus requires an organizational model for itself, the
organization for the whole will be constrained by the
need to integrate the organizations of the parts, and the
organizations of the parts will be constrained by the need
to fit into the whole.*

—RICE (1969, p. 569)

A fantasy exists that forming groups for chronically mentally ill individuals should be a straightforward task. There certainly appear to be numerous patients who would benefit from participation in group treatment. The clinician who does not carefully attend to systems and administrative issues, however, is creating roadblocks for future program development.

Social forces significantly impact upon the delivery of services to those who are least able to provide for themselves. Efforts to broaden the service delivery base have spread resources to many individuals who previously had no access to treatment. Pressures are created to "balance the budget" by limiting access or treatment provided to others. This may take the form of diminishing the size of the portal to the hospital, emergency services, or limiting a case manager's flexibility in referring clients for psychotherapeutic services. Once enrolled in a treatment setting, the type and amount of services may be limited, not only by budgetary restraints, but also by philosophical considerations. For example, the impact of changes in hospital admissions policy may have far-reaching impact. Kuhlman (1992) speculated that a series of deaths (both suicides and murders) in

51

Madison, Wisconsin, were not a random variation, but a consequence in change of admissions policy that limited access to hospital services.

The mental health system has a primary task of providing effective treatment for its patients. There are a host of subsidiary goals that include emphasizing services that the community defines as priorities, recruiting and training staff and students, and developing linkages with other appropriate agencies (Astrachan et al., 1970). There are varying pressures that may cause the organization to lose sight of its goals, and leadership is responsible for balancing and keeping in sight its tasks. This chapter will address systems elements in organizing and implementing a group program that will increase the likelihood of success.

PROGRAMMATIC CONSIDERATIONS

Administrative Elements

Administrators have to see the need for creating a group program that is compatible with their organizational goals. This may require education of those in charge regarding the therapeutic and cost benefits of a group program. Even in a situation in which there is a well-established individual treatment program for chronically ill persons, the idea of developing a comprehensive group program may appear to be beyond available resources. Therapy groups may have to be "sold" to a clinical program, keeping perspective that they represent only a portion of the overall needs of seriously mentally ill patients. How administrators will allocate limited resources is generally open to negotiation, but clinicians need to be aware of the pressures that are provoked as well as the advantages that are created with developing a group program. Programs may range from a single psychoeducational format to a more expansive program that would include walk-in groups, social skills training, and medication and process groups (these will be discussed more fully in the next section).

A fundamental cornerstone for success is a positive working alliance between clinicians and administrators. Mental health administrators have varying levels of sophistication in recognizing the necessary elements in establishing a group program, and clinicians' knowledge can be used to gain cooperation in creating the necessary clinical environment. Unforeseen difficulties are to be expected, and they require maintaining administrative collaboration as a base for problem solving.

Recruiting and Retaining Therapists

Following determination of patients' needs and formulating a plan for beginning groups, the task of developing a cadre of clinicians who are interested and committed to a group program is of primary importance. Programs suffer and fail to flourish if the leadership is not seen as endorsing the program through provision of sufficient resources and authority. Optimally, the program should be led by a senior clinician who demonstrates commitment to the program by actually conducting one or more groups.

In many settings the least experienced person is assigned to groups, with the notion that patients will take care of one another. That arrangement can create moral and organizational difficulties. Johnson and Howenstine (1982) recommended that all clinic staff assume group leadership responsibilities as part of their agreement of employment. Some find that they are not suited for this type of therapeutic endeavor and opt to discontinue their therapeutic role. However, they have had an opportunity to learn firsthand some of the advantages and pitfalls of group treatment, and consequently are in a better position to appropriately evaluate and refer patients to groups. In other settings, this procedure is not feasible. Under those circumstances, staff can be educated via case presentations or videotapes of group treatment.[1] It is obvious that educational time must be allotted for these purposes.

Training of staff should receive careful attention. Skills learned in dyadic treatment lay the groundwork for understanding individual patients, but they fall short of understanding group dynamic processes. Programs have a greater likelihood of flourishing if there are basic training and continuing education opportunities. Ongoing supervision, often in group settings, facilitates clinicians' continuing interest and skill development. Attention to the potential for staff losing interest and burning out is necessary. Solutions to this phenomenon would include perks for group therapists, which might include time and financial support to attend seminars and meetings, or importing experts who can stimulate new ideas.

Videotaping groups can serve valuable educational needs. The opportunity to review material in detail, with or without a supervisor, can be of inestimable help to observe phenomena that were not observed or understood under the pressure of the session. There are obstacles to use of videotaping. Both therapists and patients may have anxieties regarding exposure. For patients there are issues of confidentiality; for clinicians there are issues of competence. Directly addressing these issues can neutralize the fears. Providing space and equipment for videotaping is an additional, but worthwhile expense.

Educational efforts need to be extended to clinic personnel who are not conducting groups. In many settings there is a lack of sophistication about whom to refer and how to refer to groups, which results in a low referral flow. Potential candidates get lost because of staff's insufficient understanding of who might benefit from group treatment and how to get candidates into a group. Information is necessary to correct this deficit. If therapists struggle to keep group census up and must repeatedly search for members, they feel burdened and become discouraged, which increases their chances of burning out. One antidote to this process is to arrange for a group coordinator who may assume the responsibility of monitoring all of the groups in the program and determining the kinds of patients who would fit in each group. The coordinator may take on the task of conducting a brief screening interview with all group referrals (Lonergan, 1991). In that position, inappropriate candidates can be returned to the referring clinician, and appropriate candidates can be promptly referred to a group that has available space. The coordinator can also assist the group therapist(s) by providing some initial information about group treatment to the patient, as well as addressing some of the patient's anxieties.

When groups are led by cotherapists, which is the usual leadership format, regularly scheduled meetings are necessary to review the clinical work. Meetings with case managers, hospital personnel (it is inevitable that some patients will be hospitalized), or calls from emergency rooms all are time consuming. Many programs develop formulas that provide "bonus" productivity credit for the clinicians conducting groups. One such formula is for a 50% bonus credit when four or more patients attend a meeting. A requirement that eight patients attend in order for cotherapists to receive bonus credit has been viewed as too high a standard. Each administrator, working with therapists, can determine an equitable system.

The activities briefly described earlier all are time consuming. They require not only a commitment on the part of the clinician, but also that administrators allot time for these activities to take place. Not all clinicians' efforts are successful, but an atmosphere that accepts and even celebrates "good tries," can create an environment for success. In studying successful companies Peters and Waterman (1982) have observed "that the only way to succeed at all is through lots of tries, that management's primary object should be to induce lots of tries, and that a good try that results in some learning is to be celebrated even when it fails" (p. 69).

Medical Support

An important consideration in establishing a program and supporting staff is the availability of physicians to review and evaluate medications. Psychiatrists seldom directly serve as leaders, and therefore arrangements need to be firmly in place to provide the necessary medication backup. One model is for the psychiatrist to enter the group at the end of a session and review medications with the leaders present. This model, which is considered by many as optimal, simplifies communication among the treating professionals. A second model is for patients to have separate appointments that are contiguous with the meeting. This allows for more individualized attention, which might be preferable for unstable patients. A third model is to arrange for individual appointments at a time distinct from the group. This requires that patients attend the clinic on an additional occasion, but the arrangement may serve, in addition to medication checks, as an opportunity to provide brief, individualized attention to their emotional needs. Interdisciplinary collaboration results from the goodwill and respect that professionals have for one another, which are earned, not bestowed. Clinicians may have considerable satisfaction when they have established mutually respectful and supportive working alliances.

Another clinical situation arises if groups are organized to include first-episode psychotic patients or individuals who have recently been discharged from a hospital stay. These persons require considerable support to help stabilize their recovery. This may be particularly the situation with persons suffering their initial illness. In the context of more rapid discharge from hospital, many patients, their families, and other elements in the support network may require considerable support and education. The group time cannot be continually devoted to those needs and provision of additional medical/case management is in order.

Space and Staff Support

Space requirements for a large group program are considerable. Appropriate size waiting rooms and group rooms are necessary. A luxury might be a sufficiently large group room to enable restless or agitated patients an opportunity to leave the group circle without having to leave the meeting room. A place in the room for a coffee pot provides for oral gratification, and a sanctioned way for a patients to temporarily relieve tension and leave the group without exiting the room.

Paperwork documenting patients' treatment can be a significant burden. In keeping with the ideology of group treatment, meeting records should be in the form of a group note, rather than individual progress notes. A viable solution has been dictation of a group process note (of course, necessitating secretarial support) that is then duplicated and placed in each member's record. Patients are identified by first names and last initials, thereby preserving anonymity of others to a reasonable extent. All those present should be mentioned in the process note, even if it is merely an observation about nonverbal behavior or a member's silence throughout the meeting.

A characteristic of working with chronically ill individuals is that many individuals attend treatment erratically. Patients will respond to efforts encouraging them to come to meetings after they have missed appointments. Secretarial staff may routinely send reminders to patients of their appointments or contact patients who have missed sessions. Such reminders serve to increase attendance and maintain the program (Chen, 1991).

Events within the clinic that impact upon the treatment staff, although they do not directly affect a group or its members, nevertheless may reverberate through the group. For example, a favored receptionist may lose her job, or a new telephone operator may mix up messages. Kibel (1990) writes, "Given that these [inpatients] are overdependent on external objects, analytic investigation of their pathology should be conducted in a social context" (p. 247). Awareness of situations that may represent change or deprivation will enable therapists to understand patients' associations and their anxieties. Clinicians also are subjected to clinic-wide events that may impact upon their functioning.

> *Example*: A psychiatrist, whose contract with the clinic was not renewed, angrily departed without telling his patients that he was leaving. That task was left to the new caretakers. One of the cotherapists was a senior administrator, who had been held responsible for the physician's termination. The other cotherapist, a resident, was quite saddened by the psychiatrist's departure. Only a single group member had direct contact with the psychiatrist, but his departure had reverberated through the clinic.
>
> In the first group session after the psychiatrist's termination, one patient wondered about the psychiatrist's absence, which was followed by a question about the resident leaving the group—the members knew she would depart in 6 months, at the end of the academic year. Another member said he was leaving the city.
>
> The following week, the patients spent the entire session talking about parents and children. It never became clear whether parents caused children to be sick, or whether children acted up and caused their parents difficulty.

In discussing these sessions in supervision, the therapists failed to make a linkage between the two meetings. When the connection was pointed out as the patients' metaphorical feelings about departing therapists, countertransferences were explored. The cotherapist administrator was startled at herself for not making the connection, but readily commented on her wish that the entire episode of the dismissed psychiatrist would go away. The resident cotherapist said that she found herself thinking concretely, rather than utilizing her usual capacity to hear metaphors, and that she had been pained by the departure of the psychiatrist. Thus the system issue impacted in a major way on several meetings, affecting not only the members, but also the clinicians.

Many of the administrative considerations require staff or clinician time and therefore diminish the cost effectiveness of group treatment. On balance, there remains a cost efficiency, because therapist time is seldom lost because of the failure of all patients to attend a scheduled meeting. In addition, once a group program is established and running, clinicians develop considerable loyalty to the treatment format and genuinely enjoy their work.

TYPES OF GROUPS

A spectrum of groups exists that serve a variety of therapeutic needs. Waiting rooms provide opportunities for socialization, and the interaction may be augmented by providing refreshments and a volunteer host. Slightly more structured opportunities for patient interaction are social clubs. These are ancillary to the more formal modalities but can serve a useful function in enlarging patients' opportunities for socialization, and they may make attending other treatments more attractive.

The following is a brief description of the more common group formats employed in working with chronically ill persons.

Psychoeducational Groups

Psychoeducational groups are time-limited approaches designed to provide information about specific illnesses to patients or significant others. The hypothesis underlying these groups is the existence of a biological basis of many chronic illnesses. Attendees are given lectures, shown films, provided literature, and offered opportunities to raise questions in a generally didactic/discussion format. The goals of these groups are primarily to educate individuals and others about the nature and course of an illness. Specifics regarding the known biology help reduce family guilt about "causing" the illness, and efforts are made, particularly for families of schizophrenic individuals, to educate them about the impact of expressed emotion on relapse. Treatment alternatives are outlined, so that patients and families may make informed choices regarding their options. Included in these discussions is information regarding the range of medications, their therapeutic benefits, and side effects. The clinical course of the illness is described, with a goal of clarifying early signs of relapse and the role of early intervention in preventing or delaying increased impairment.

In addition, the dynamics of psychoeducational groups allow participants to identify with one another, decreasing stigmatization and isolation. Knowledge of the course of the illness often alters negative expectations of continuing morbidity and instills hope. Social linkages made in psychoeducational sessions may be continued outside the meetings, thereby increasing the generally diminished social network of the chronically ill.

Psychoeducational groups are usually limited from 6 to 12 sessions. Leaders need to have a thorough knowledge of the educational material and have access to appropriate resources that will fill in the inevitable gaps in knowledge.

Social Skills Training Groups

Social skills training has been useful to help individuals overcome interpersonal deficits that interfere with their daily functioning. Behavioral and learning strategies are applied to specified problems, and patients may practice them within the group through role playing. Therapists praise patients' accomplishments in order to reinforce effective behaviors. In this atmosphere, corrective feedback is given. Specific problems such as making eye contact, speaking directly, asserting oneself, or approaching strangers might be addressed. Patients are given homework assignments to reinforce and generalize the learning. In some programs, patients are accompanied into the community where the practiced skills are applied *in vivo*.

Therapists are active, directive, and help patients define specific behavioral tasks. However, schizophrenic patients appear to have difficulty generalizing gains or sustaining them, particularly in the absence of continuing contact with the clinician.

Walk-In Groups

Walk-in groups have achieved some measure of success. They serve as supplements to emergency-type services and can become part of the fabric of a clinic. Patients may attend the group at any scheduled meeting and discuss either crises or ongoing problems. These groups meet the needs of a subgroup of the chronic population that is unwilling or unable to commit to a more structured format. When necessary, such groups may be used to provide medications with a minimum of administrative red tape.

Group cohesion does not develop to a significant degree. Instead, the focus is primarily on individual problem solving in a group setting. Others do gain from hearing problems and potentially sharing some of their own concerns, but the major thrust of these groups is their function as a useful stopgap.

Walk-in groups only slowly gain credibility, in part because initial attendance is variable and often low. Over a period of time, the groups can develop a patient "following" that is sufficient to justify a clinician's time. The groups often are subject to criticism for not satisfactorily meeting patients' needs. They can provide an alternative for patients in crises who may need an extra appointment or for persons who seldom keep scheduled appointments. However, from many patients' perspectives, such groups are insufficient to meet their needs.

Clinicians also are prone to burnout, and often the least sophisticated therapists are assigned as leaders. Rotation of leaders on a schedule is one solution to the burnout problem. Collaboration between individual and group therapists is essential to minimize conflict and to share the responsibilities of care for these individuals.

Medication Groups

Medication groups have become very popular as a method of providing an opportunity for social interaction and a regular schedule for patients to renew their medications. For patients who are resistant to exploring their life situation or merely wish limited contact, medication groups fulfill an important need. Program designs range from providing a waiting room where volunteers promote interaction while patients are waiting to be seen for medication, to a session in which medications or problems in living are discussed. Many of the groups described in the historical review fit in this category. Dynamics of these groups serve to provide some interaction, but topics often focus on medications and their side effects. Examination of relationships generally is not a high priority. Patients can be given a specific appointment to return, thereby providing some structure.

These groups can be quite large, with a census of 25–30 individuals. Scheduling enables the clinic to limit the expected number of patients to attend each week. Provision of refreshments in the form of snacks and coffee or other beverages is frequently part of this model. Patients generally are scheduled for monthly or bimonthly sessions. Coleadership is commonly advocated. In some groups, patients are called out of the room to discuss their medication and then may return to the group following this intervention. In other groups, patients merely return to their prior activities following receipt of medication.

Psychiatrists are involved with prescribing medication, but rarely serve as clinicians during the group interaction. This is a popular model in which nurses serve as group clinicians, because they are familiar with medication effects.

Time-Limited Groups

Time-limited groups represent a treatment model addressing specific problems in the context of continuing pharmacotherapy. The model advocated by Kanas et al. (1989a) addresses schizophrenic patients' specific problems of hallucinations, disordered thinking (paranoid or grandiose ideas), and social isolation. In a semistructured format, members are asked to share their experiences, and each individual is addressed regarding the problem under discussion. After eliciting information from each member, the therapist inquires about patients' coping strategies: for example, "How do you handle the voices that you hear?"

The goals of these groups are to diminish patients' feelings of isolation in relation to their symptoms, finding ways of coping with psychotic material, and learning strategies for improving social relationships.

The groups are co-led, may include from 6 to 10 individuals, are of 45–60 minutes' duration, and are limited to 10–12 sessions. Patients are recruited following hospitalization or from medication clinics. Upon completion of the prescribed number of sessions, they are referred back to their treating clinician to continue their medication and other indicated treatment.

Process Groups

Process groups can be focused mainly on providing supportive treatment, or they may have an additional goal of patients' gaining understanding of their own contribution to their social adjustment. At times, linkages are made to historical experiences that can provide insight into current behaviors. The following is only a brief description of the nature of these groups.

All treatment groups strive to provide support. The common element is an effort to create a degree of group cohesion, in which members can feel a sense of belonging and freedom to express themselves. Therapists make linkages between and among members, thereby decreasing isolation. Universalization of problems, decreasing the perceived boundaries between health and illness, addressing the impairments caused by the illness or the societal response to being mentally ill are elements that contribute to members' engagement in the group. Sharing problem-solving strategies, or addressing painful feelings (particularly neglect, isolation, loneliness, and rejection) are major therapeutic aims.

In some groups, behavioral techniques are utilized. Patients may be asked to rehearse specific roles in anticipation of situations in their lives, for example, a job interview or a drug-abusing relative.

Some process groups shift to helping patients develop insight into their own contributions to their problems. Therapists directly translate metaphorical associations into the here and now of the group, in contrast to more supportive strategies in which metaphors are addressed in the displacement. Intragroup transactions are explored (to the extent of the members' abilities) in relation to boundary alterations (e.g., absences or changes of members or leaders), and responses to the therapists (transferences) and to peers. Positive and supportive peer interaction is present in almost all process groups, but sexual and aggressive feelings are generally eschewed. It is these latter feelings that are addressed in groups geared toward working at greater depth.

Membership in process groups may be homogeneous or heterogeneous by diagnosis. Process groups are generally of 45–75 minutes' duration, although in some settings a traditional 90-minute time frame is used. Efforts are made to ensure that five to eight members are present for each meeting, although the group roster may be larger because of patients' proclivities not to attend all sessions.

Programs may utilize several of these modalities in their overall work with the chronically mentally ill. It is important, however, to specify the type of group that is planned and determine if there is sufficient administrative support.

SUMMARY

In this chapter, the tasks of initiating a group program have been examined. Clinicians need to attend to administrative considerations and the politics of the clinic setting. An effective administrative alliance increases the potential for success.

Attention to the special resources required to sustain a program pays dividends in assuring its success. Among the considerations are arrangements for patients' medication, and concrete elements of space, secretarial support, and methods aimed at minimizing the necessary paperwork. Moreover, attention to the needs of the group therapists helps sustain their interest and prevent staff burnout and turnover.

A variety of groups serving this population's needs can be established, and they can be viewed as complementary, rather than competitive. All have a place in assisting subpopulations of chronically ill patients.

SEVEN

THERAPEUTIC GOALS
AND SUPPORTIVE TREATMENT

> *Less "psychologically minded" persons who need us just*
> *as badly are seen as less desirable patients, are less apt to*
> *be taken into therapy, and may sense in some way that*
> *they are second choice.*
>
> —LAMB (1986, p. 869)

Treatment goals for chronically mentally ill persons vary considerably, as they do for any other segment of the mentally ill population. It is a gross oversimplification for therapists to limit their tasks to providing support, stabilization, and adjustment because a portion of the chronically ill population has the capacity to make considerable changes. Those latter individuals recover, disappear from mental health networks and are absorbed into the community, often functioning without any formal therapeutic contacts. Harding and her colleagues (1987b) reported on a startling positive outcome for schizophrenic patients, many of whom had been hospitalized for extended periods. Such outcomes run counter to popular wisdom. This chapter will examine treatment goals in the framework of group psychotherapy.

For many seriously and continuing ill individuals, safe housing, food, or medical care are of higher priority than care of their emotional disabilities (Lehman, 1983; Mechanic & Aiken, 1987). A degree of environmental stability is necessary before engaging individuals in treatment that requires attendance at a specified time and place. It may be beyond clinicians' expertise or interest to assist patients in obtaining such services, but it behooves them to be aware of how to help individuals obtain assistance in these sectors of their lives. Understanding impediments to attending treatment seems fundamental, and considerations such as providing bus tokens or arranging treatment times that fit with bus schedules or do not interfere with mealtimes in room-and-board homes make a difference in attendance. If therapists limit their therapeutic focus to intrapsychic or interpersonal dynamics, the reality elements in patients' lives may be neglected.

An accurate and complete diagnosis, including information about medical illness, becomes the basis for goal setting. Substance abuse is such a frequent concomitant of chronic mental illness that particular efforts should be made to assess drugs' contribution to a person's illness. Many treatment programs establish a goal of abstinence or control of addiction before placing individuals in a group. Relapse is not infrequent, and managing the slip may temporarily take precedence over other treatment considerations.

Medical illnesses are quite prevalent among mentally ill persons. They have difficulty gaining access to a medical system that provides continuity of care. Acute medical illnesses are often treated in emergency settings, and less acute but chronic illnesses are frequently neglected. Therapists need to maintain awareness of the whole person in the process of addressing psychosocial processes.

Optimally, goals are established as a collaborative effort between patient and therapist. Generally, a period of negotiation is necessary to arrive at mutually acceptable treatment goals. Nevertheless, some chronically ill individuals enter therapy at the recommendation of their referral source and compliantly accept the clinician's recommendation without articulating their own treatment wishes. Under these circumstances, goals are primarily established by the therapist. They should reflect an understanding of patients' assets and liabilities, life circumstances, social networks, and psychodynamics.

Patients' psychodynamics strongly influence what changes can be expected and therefore the treatment goals. Internal conflicts and developmental arrests limit patients' abilities to use their innate capacities. Appreciation of individuals' life histories and interactional patterns, their anxieties and their fears, as well as their hopes and wishes, enables clinicians to monitor "small changes." This knowledge has a predictive component, because dynamic understanding will enable therapists to recognize common inner meanings of seemingly dissimilar situations. Informing patients of potential triggers to stress or helping them understand common threads in apparently disparate events can prevent decompensation and increase their capacities to manage their lives.

TREATMENT GOALS

The long-established goal in analytic psychotherapy has been increased self-awareness and self-understanding—in analytic parlance, insight. At times, insight has been elevated to a superordinate position, eschewing behavioral change. Other forms of therapeutic intervention place behavioral change as the highest priority. Behavioral methods, cognitive restructuring, and medications are aimed at target symptoms or behaviors. Accumulated wisdom transcends ideological boundaries, and technical innovations are utilized in helping to overcome the multidimensional elements in working with the chronically mentally ill.

Treatment goals are usefully linked to the stage of illness. Following a period of decompensation, which might include hospitalization, the primary goal is restabilization. This is particularly salient in an era of brief hospital stays in which generally only the most acute symptoms are resolved. Attention to continuation of medications and to the environment, including basic survival and social needs takes priority. In circumstances following recompensation from an acute illness, Breier and Strauss (1984) succinctly observed that "the character of social relationships in the convalescent phase tended to be one-sided and dependent, the patients asking much from the relationships and seeming to have little to give" (p. 953). Goals should be concordant with patients' needs, and therapists should refrain from prematurely pressuring patients to return to work or attempt relationships that would be expected to be mutually satisfying.

After stabilizing, patients are more likely to reinvest in reciprocal social relationships, consider longer term life plans, or express curiosity about the causes and consequences of their illness. Therapeutic goals may then shift to take into account changes in patients' capacities. Many individuals are not interested in gaining self-understanding and are more prone to seal over the experience of their acute illness (McGlashan et al., 1975).

For persons expressing an interest in gaining insight into themselves, it is important to recognize that self-awareness is multidimensional and includes global appreciation of the disorder, effects of medication in changing mental states, social consequences of the illness in the present and past, and the presence of thought disorder (Amador et al., 1993). Schizophrenic patients have less awareness of having a mental disorder than individuals diagnosed with schizoaffective disorder, major depressive disorder, or major depressive disorder with psychosis (Amador et al., 1994). Deficits in awareness include symptoms, social consequences of the illness, and effects of medication. The diminished awareness is apparently a trait and is not state dependent. Patients in remission do not differ from those in acute exacerbation. Insight into triggers for anxiety, stress tolerance, or inner conflicts shifts the therapeutic emphasis from insight into interpersonal relations to aspects of intrapsychic functioning.

Optimally, patients and therapists establish goals that are mutually acceptable. This may be more difficult to achieve during a decompensated phase of illness, in which the clinician's knowledge of consequences of behaviors may require action that the patient does not agree with. However, as the illness stabilizes and becomes more chronic, a collaborative relationship increases chances for achieving desired goals.

INTERPERSONAL DYNAMICS

Fundamental to understanding patients' interpersonal transactions in the group setting is an appreciation of their intrapsychic developmental needs, conflicts, and arrests that interfere with their ability to enter into comfortable and productive exchanges. Dynamics can be conceptualized around tasks of developing trust, resolving dependency needs, managing separation–individuation, and consolidating reliable self-boundaries.

A basic sense of trust in oneself and in others is essential for optimal psychological growth. Experiences of many continually ill persons can be linked to serious deficits in their capacity to form trusting relationships. A variety of character formations and defenses may be employed for self-protection. Often patients exhibit efforts at control, such as failure to attend treatment, monopolization, critical attacks on others, or use of idiosyncratic language as manifestations of failures in forming trusting relationships.

Developmental failures interfere with patients' capacity to maintain their inner equilibrium in the face of situations in which their trust in others is disrupted. In this context, patients distrust their abilities to constrain their responses, and consequently they may resort to a variety of self-soothing activities, including use of drugs and alcohol. Angry or enraged outbursts may represent patients' efforts to distance themselves from hurtful situations, or their response may be a communication to others to desist from noxious behavior.

Development of trust that one will be responded to in an empathic manner and the capacity to suffer narcissistic injury without internal disruption are not limited to early childhood experiences. They are also products of interactions at all developmental stages. Children in latency and adolescence, who are "peculiar" because of biological–genetic factors, frequently experience peer ostracism or rejection. They become very cautious in expressing themselves, which may lead to further alienation. Xenophobia, in all of its overt and subtle forms, contributes to rejection of others, which may exacerbate a downward spiral of distrust.

Closely associated with experiences of basic trust are those of dependency. For some individuals developmental thrusts to explore the world have been severely inhibited. Careful historical reconstruction will often reveal a disturbed child–parent relationship. Images of clinging, demanding, or engulfing persons are hallmarks of severely unmet dependency needs. Some individuals exhibit dependent behaviors beginning in the initial stages of a relationship, whereas others will enact those needs when they have developed sufficient trust in another person.

The stage of separation–individuation may be characterized by alternate clinging dependent behavior and pseudoindependence. Inconsistencies emerge in which patients exhibit mature interactions, only to respond to stress with rapid regression and reemergence of previously explored and temporarily mastered immature behaviors. At times patients become dependent without consciously recognizing how meaningful others have become to them, and only under the pressure of a member's departure or a treatment interruption (which may be the result of either the patient's or the clinician's absence) do these dynamics clearly emerge. An individual's capacity to be alone and to tolerate aloneness is a crucial developmental achievement. For patients to acquire inner stability in the face of loss may require extended periods of treatment.

Attainment of stable self-boundaries is a significant developmental step. Mutually satisfying relationships require individuals to open personal boundaries without fearing that they will be unable to close them again. In groups, a frequent manifestation of boundary instability is members' suppression of discussion of others' illness or symptoms out of fear of emotional contagion. Subgrouping, either inside or outside the meeting, is a strategy that protects against boundaries being overwhelmed by the group mass. At times abrupt/premature terminations are expressions of patients' fears of losing themselves in the group.

Supportive treatment interventions are based on understanding the developmental arrests and regressive potentials of seriously mentally ill individuals and have been aimed at stabilizing and supporting their adaptation to their environment.

SUPPORTIVE THERAPY

Supportive therapy has long been relegated to a secondary position in the multitude of dynamic insight–reconstructive forms of therapeutic intervention. In part, this status is due to inadequate differentiation between support as a treatment goal based on patients' disabilities and support as a technique, which is intrinsic to every therapeutic encounter. An additional salient distinction is that of treating the illness and treating the ill person (Minkoff & Stern, 1985). Many chronic mental illnesses have a biological component, and in a distortion of the tradition of medicine, the illness is treated and the individual is relatively neglected. A balance is necessary between individual and illness perspectives.

The concepts of supportive treatment are broadly based. When supportive goals and strategies are integrated within a psychodynamic framework, clinicians are in a better position to anticipate the impact of a particular intervention and to track its therapeutic value. Although not a specific technique, among the most useful supportive elements is the clinician's capacity to remain with patients over extended periods, often encompassing years. The presence of a steady person, who has been with the chronically ill patient through successes and failures and has been able to maintain interest and caring, is stabilizing and growth enhancing.

Supportive Goals

For chronically ill individuals, therapeutic goals may be conceptualized as providing treatment that will enable patients to remain in the community, find satisfaction in their daily lives, and increase their capacity to adapt to ordinary stresses of living. Nevertheless, specific goals shift across time. For instance, decompensating patients, who have discontinued their medication, may require encouragement to take their drugs in order to prevent further disorganization and hospitalization. Under these circumstances, techniques will focus on the illness and efforts to contain the exacerbation of the acute symptoms. Yet each individual's specific personal resources must be taken into account in order to achieve a goal of stabilizing an illness. Similarly, recently discharged patients may require therapeutic strategies that promote stabilization before addressing adaptation (Breier & Strauss, 1984).

Supportive treatment goals have been variously defined. Novalis et al. (1993, p. 7) list frequent goals of supportive psychotherapy:

- Reducing behavioral dysfunctions
- Reducing subjective mental distress
- Supporting and enhancing the patient's strengths and coping skills, and his or her capacity to use environmental supports
- Maximizing treatment autonomy
- Achieving maximum possible independence from psychiatric illness

Goals are not limited to these elements, and less frequent goals would include patients' gaining self-understanding of their interpersonal experiences or inner emotional life. Indeed, instructing a decompensating patient on the necessity of resumption of taking medication may not only reduce behavioral dysfunction, but also serves to begin a process in which a patient might gain insight into the reasons for stopping medication. This might include exploration of the patient's decision to stop, which may have been based on unreported, unacceptable side effects. The path may then lead to gaining an understanding of the patient's reluctance to report the difficulty and a host of dynamic issues, such as the need to act independently, fear of being misunderstood, or mistrust of clinicians.

Decisions about specific goals are based on patients' capacities as delineated through careful exploration of individuals' histories and unfolding of behaviors in relation to the clinician and the treatment process. Assessment optimally would include the following:

- Delineation of developmental achievements
- Coping capacities
- Management of anxiety and aggression (as representatives of affective stimulation)
- Acceptance of affection and intimacy (in part reflections of basic trust)
- Ability for self-reflection
- Intellectual capacities
- Motivation to change

Motivation is particularly difficult to define, because patients tend to protect themselves from being emotionally traumatized, and only in a setting where they can accumulate evidence that they will not be injured will they expose deeper motivations and express willingness to take risks leading to change. These are seldom easy evaluations, and patients will often behave in contradictory and ambiguous manners that complicate assessment. A neglected element in determining motivation is directly inquiring what the patient wishes for and hopes to achieve. Certainly the potential for success is enhanced when therapeutic goals are mutually agreed upon.

Buckley (1986, p. 516) lists dynamic indications for supportive therapy:

- Predomination of primitive impulses
- Impairment of object relations
- Inadequate modulation of affect
- Overwhelming anxiety around separation–individuation issues

In addition, persons with major deficits in reality testing or preoccupation with somatic symptoms often are candidates for supportive treatment.

These various guidelines serve to inform clinicians that careful evaluation and individual assessment are necessary before making a determination of appropriate goals.

Supportive Techniques

Techniques of supportive therapy are in the service of achieving treatment goals. Support is intrinsic to all treatment endeavors and creates a sense of safety or a holding environment. Of major significance is the patient's *experience* of support, because interventions made by a clinician or group members might not accurately fit with the person's needs and might have an unanticipated noxious impact. For example, ill-timed reassurances are commonly received as others' efforts to suppress feelings and have the effect of shutting down and further alienating patients, rather than calming them. Unfortunately, patients seldom directly voice their responses to such experiences.

The degree of clinician activity is a central element in supportive techniques. Patients are continually scrutinizing their therapists to determine their degree of interest. Many chronically ill patients equate silence with disinterest, and they experience aloneness. Extended periods of silence promote patients' shifting their attention from group interactions to inner processes or fantasies about external experiences. A patient's capacity to tolerate being alone is tested by periods of silence and may result in the emergence of regressive behaviors or symptoms. In the transference, silence may represent neglect or ostracism. Activity may take the form of asking questions or linking the silence to the immediately preceding treatment process, or to prior discussions that reflected the same theme. However, a stereotyped inquiry, "What is happening in the group?," may be experienced as disinterest or as nonhuman. An example of linking might be, "We were also talking about feelings of stigmatization several weeks ago, and you, Joan, had some thoughts about managing it. Does what we were just discussing seem similar to you or to others?"

Therapist activity should not preclude the crucial capacity to respectfully listen and to respond. Creating a setting in which patients can freely ventilate feelings and in which they are recognized for their achievements and efforts at problem solving has considerable therapeutic benefit. Listening should not be seen as equivalent to agreement, because to merely hear about self-defeating behaviors may reflect a countertransference. Reassurance and praise (in its various forms) must be provided when the situation actually warrants such a response. In most circumstances, new behaviors are undertaken with a degree of ambivalence, and patients can be reassured that they are not unique (universalization) in having mixed feelings—"I am aware that even though you were pleased that you stood your ground with your mother, as with most people, there is also a part of you that feared she would get upset and become angry with you." Such an intervention addresses patients' sense of themselves as well as indicating that they are not different from others because of their feelings. It bolsters patients' awareness that their own feelings are valuable. More direct support can be provided with comments such as "I agree with your response."

Advice may assist patients in becoming unstuck and finding more useful alternatives. Advice should be provided from the patient's perspective and might include several alternatives. For example, "You have often found visiting your mother upsetting. Would it be easier for you to tell her in advance you can only stay for one hour?" Framing advice in this fashion engages the patient in collaborative problem solving.

More active supportive techniques include role playing and setting up scenarios of problem situations in which the patient can practice alternative strategies in the therapeutic setting. These behavioral techniques can be integrated into dynamic supportive treatment, but the clinician needs to keep in mind that patients may have important unspoken emotional responses to the explicit control that often accompanies use of these strategies. For example, a group member may transferentially react to the proposal to role play as a repetition of parental domination.

Therapist self-disclosure, which is often used when the clinician wishes to illustrate an alternative way of managing a difficult situation, should be open to constant self-scrutiny. The potential for countertransference, particularly in the sector of exhibitionism, is ever present. Moreover, self-disclosure in the context of the therapist's wishing to illustrate alternative responses to situations may be suggesting solutions that are beyond patients' capacities at that time. Therapeutic ambition may override assessment of patients' capacities. Answering questions about oneself can be given within social conventions of privacy and reticence (Winston et al., 1986). Patients often wish for answers from the therapist's experience, thereby creating considerable pull to fulfill the role of expert, perhaps in areas beyond the clinician's own experiences. We are all susceptible to self-aggrandizement.

Supportive interventions may not have their intended salutary effect. Patients respond as they attach meaning to the interventions in concert with their own life experiences. For instance, a comment that was intended to be empathic and soothing may result in associations to being intruded upon or controlled. By attending to patients' responses, most frequently as metaphors, therapists will gain a window into the impact of their comments. It behooves the clinician to be open to hearing patients' negative responses to what was intended to be supportive and helpful.

Group Therapeutic Factors and Support

Dynamic interactions in therapeutic groups provide support for members in ways that differ from those available in dyadic treatment. MacKenzie (1990), modifying the pioneering work of Yalom (1970), suggests that group therapeutic factors may be placed in four clusters:

> *Supportive factors*
> > Acceptance
> > Universality
> > Instillation of hope
> > Altruism
>
> *Self-revelation factors*
> > Self-disclosure
> > Catharsis
>
> *Learning from others*
> > Modeling
> > Vicarious learning
> > Guidance
> > Education
>
> *Psychological work factors*
> > Self-understanding
> > Interpersonal input
> > Interpersonal output

Supportive factors assume considerable importance for seriously ill patients who have diminished social networks. The presence of peers who are interested and responsive to a member's problems expands the universe of those who are accepting of the patient. Emphasizing the special meaning of peers are the members' observations that they pay the therapist to listen to them, but fellow members respond because they care.

Acceptance does not automatically accrue with membership but develops through interactions. In newly forming groups, members, in general, cautiously test to determine if they will be accepted. Being responded to in a positive, understanding manner facilitates trust and leads to greater self-revelation, which also requires understanding. A positive therapeutic spiral may ensue.

Some individuals exhibit their pathology very early, either verbally or behaviorally. These responses represent difficult management problems, because such individuals are very familiar with rejection and only faintly hope that they might be accepted despite their difficulties. A groupwide norm of acceptance (but not passive masochism) can be very facilitating to newcomers who may anticipate psychological disaster as the price for joining a group. The new member may stimulate memories of how each veteran joined. Their reminiscences serve to decrease a new member's sense of isolation and promote universality, which is an interlocking supportive element.

Universalization arises from several sources. Patients tell their stories, and they can identify with one another, thereby decreasing their sense of aloneness. Moreover, they observe reflections of their own behaviors in others' interactions. This mirroring is an additional source of linking. A particularly salient element in universalization processes is accomplished through sharing of experiences and affects about stigmatization. Patients share experiences of family, friends, or prospective employers' aversive responses to learning that they have had a serious mental illness requiring continued treatment. It is a rare patient who does not participate in such discussions.

Groups provide a source of hope, which is a powerful supportive element. Members' notice others making changes that may have seemed unattainable, and they observe others managing frustrations in interpersonal exchanges with family members or strangers, in finding new problem-solving strategies, or in obtaining part-time or full-time work. Observations of colleagues' successes not only provide hope but also serve as a source for imitation or identification.

Group membership creates opportunities for patients to be helpful to one another. When this takes place without the expectation of reciprocity, the process is labeled "altruism." A person's sense of personal efficacy is enhanced when his or her idea or suggestion proves to be useful to another. Chronically ill individuals have wide-ranging experiences with a multitude of bureaucracies. They know the ins and outs of obtaining housing, transportation, or other forms of assistance that may be unknown to clinicians. Patients' pleasure in seeing others benefit from shared information is palpable, and observing the value of their suggestions functions to increase self-esteem. Within the treatment setting, patients' capacities to ask useful questions or make observations about one another add to feelings of self-worth and to a belief that participating in group treatment is worthwhile.

Being helpful is not limited to interactions taking place within the treatment setting. Chronically ill patients are not tightly restrained to limit outside contacts among members. They frequently make contact with one another by phone, meet to come to the sessions together, or may extend the sessions by postgroup socializing. These meetings may expand into genuine, enduring friendships. At times, they may be life saving, as illustrated by a patient experiencing chest pains of a heart attack and phoning a fellow member who helped get him to the hospital. Clearly, the sense of therapeutic community and support extends beyond the consultation room for this population.

Supportive factors may stand alone in the treatment process. However, they are also building blocks for other therapeutic factors. Self-revelation factors of self-disclosure and catharsis overlap with supportive elements. Patients in a position of emotional support are more prepared to learn from others and delve into psychological work. Patients may respond to feedback with insight into their psychodynamics (Bloch & Crouch, 1985). Illustrative of one level of insight was a schizophrenic patient who regularly received injectable antipsychotic medication. In the meeting, she observed that she was talking too much because she had neglected to get her regularly scheduled shot the previous week. Another example was a dependent, mildly retarded man who learned that his semiautomatic expression, "I'm finished," was an indicator that he had become upset with the situation he was describing. Others learn about themselves through the relationships that they form with members outside the group and bring back for discussion. They may learn that they have expectations that others are not likely to meet. This process is facilitated when both parties are present and an opportunity is provided to hear all sides of a conflict.

Patients may develop intellectualized understanding of some developmental events that have contributed to their illness. Although insights are rarely in-depth, patients feel a sense of mastery in providing explanations of their behaviors.

> *Example*: A very difficult, monopolizing woman with schizoaffective illness, after many months, came to understand that she was very frightened of being placed in the role of caring for the other members, as she had by her mother, who used her to care for 10 younger siblings. She observed that certain things triggered her feelings, and her response was like the cap coming off the volcano. This metaphor was then used to support the patient in gaining self-control and altered a group atmosphere in which she felt suppressed and not understood.

Similar learning may take place vicariously as others talk about adverse life experiences.

Members' experiences of support from peers may serve to counteract the clinician's therapeutic optimism or pessimism, thereby balancing the treatment process. They become quite capable of soothing one another in the face of the therapist's inevitable misunderstandings.

Therapists and patients perspectives differ regarding therapeutic factors. Training may influence what clinicians consider important. Indeed, if patients do not readily verbalize their inner states, report changes in their lives, or demonstrate new behaviors in the treatment setting, the clinician is hard put to identify the impact of treatment. Nevertheless, inner change may be taking place. As reported by Bloch and Crouch (1985), "Therapists may be more inclined to focus on observed behavior than to hazard guesses about their patients' inner experiences, while patients can report subjective phenomena, such as new insights, learning from fellow group members and feeling hopeful about improvement" (p. 228).

Empirical studies assessing therapeutic factors sampling seriously ill individuals has been limited. Yalom (1985) reviewed studies of hospitalized patients and found that instillation of hope and assumption of responsibility (existential factors operationalized in research as "assumption of ultimate responsibility for my own life" [p. 106]) "loomed large" in hospitalized patients' ratings of therapeutic factors. Day treatment patients rated group cohesiveness highest among the therapeutic factors, in contrast to outpatients, who rated self-understanding highest (Butler & Fuhriman, 1980). Macaskill (1982) reported that hospitalized borderline women rated self-understanding and altruism as the most helpful factors in their group treatment. However, he also asked respondents to provide an illustrative example to ascertain if they understood the questions. When the responses were examined, Macaskill concluded that patients responded to questions pertaining to self-understanding as "holding communications, and the therapist was perceived as providing good-enough mothering" (p. 68). As this report illustrates, studies are difficult to evaluate, because patients interpret items on research questionnaires in seemingly idiosyncratic ways.

SUMMARY

This chapter has explored the therapeutic task of establishing treatment goals that are acceptable to patients and are compatible with their assets and liabilities. The fundamental importance of making an accurate and thorough diagnosis, which would include psychosocial considerations, is stressed. Attention is drawn to the salience of exploring for chemical dependency and physical illness in this vulnerable population.

Interpersonal dynamics reflect intrapsychic development and conflict. Dynamics of chronically mentally ill individuals will center on issues of trust, dependency, separation–individuation, and boundary building.

Supportive therapy provides for the needs of this population and is compatible with many individuals' treatment goals. Indications and techniques of supportive treatment are examined and placed in the context of therapeutic factors emanating from a group treatment format.

EIGHT

FORMING THE GROUP

The term "group therapy" can have two meanings. It can refer to the treatment of a number of individuals assembled for special therapeutic sessions, or it can refer to a planned endeavor to develop in a group the forces that lead to smoothly running co-operative activity.

—BION (1961, p. 11)

In this chapter, the practical elements involved in forming dynamically oriented groups for chronically mentally ill patients will be addressed. The major tasks are deciding on the group organization, composition, recruiting, interviewing, and preparing patients. In addition, the clinician will find it necessary to maintain relationships with others in the system in order to ensure a continuing referral base. Attention to the administrative considerations of appropriate support for space, clerical assistance, linkages to other components of care (case management, medication management), clinician support, and sustenance have been examined in Chapter 6.

Many of these tasks are more readily managed if there is a commitment to developing a group program within the mental health center. The advantages of starting multiple groups are considerable: There is a sharing of interest and support among clinicians; more than one or two therapists will be considering referrals; the intake processes for patients entering into the system will be more attuned to considering group treatment; and the tendency to sequester and isolate a particular treatment modality will be diminished.

GROUP ORGANIZATION

The organization of the group should be decided on in conjunction with its composition and goals. In keeping with an overall goal of providing stabilization and opportunities for growth, groups should be organized to continue indefinitely and have no planned termination. Hogarty (1993), working with schizophrenic patients in family treatment and in social skills training, observes; "Thus it appears . . . that when treatment ends, its effects end" (p. 22). Similarly, depression with its propensity for relapse often requires continuing, but possibly less intense treatment (Klerman & Weissman, 1992).

Groups for the seriously mentally ill generally meet for briefer time periods than comparable groups composed of neurotic or higher level personality-disordered patients. Sessions lasting 45–75 minutes are generally of sufficient length. A useful structure provides segments of 45–60 minutes for process and 15 minutes for medication review. Members may leave or remain during the latter segment. If a physician is not leading the group, the person responsible for managing medication may enter during this period and in the presence of the therapist(s) make any necessary medication adjustments. This procedure simplifies communication among the responsible clinicians and does not require patients to make separate clinic visits.

Generally, groups are scheduled to meet weekly. Less frequent bi-weekly or monthly formats are faced with a problem of continuity when the schedule is disrupted for holidays or therapists' absence. Groups established primarily for medication renewal and support may be scheduled to meet on a monthly basis. This schedule may be effective if similar groups meet at the same time during the other weeks, and therapists have sufficient flexibility to allow patients to attend another group if their meeting is canceled. A flexible multigroup format also allows patients to be seen more frequently if they are under stress or experiencing an exacerbation of major symptoms. Such an option is more readily applicable if the groups are led by the same clinician (Seeman, 1981).

Membership rosters range from 12–18 persons. In most groups, the core member subgroup varies from three to six individuals (de Bosset, 1988). Others attend either irregularly or on a fixed but less frequent basis. Optimally, weekly participation should be in the range of six to nine individuals. The roster may be smaller when initiating a group, but continuing attention must be paid to recruiting members in order to maintain a satisfactory census. A flow chart plotting weekly attendance serves as a useful reminder of shifting overall participation patterns. Many groups have slow attrition rates or experience moderate fluctuations in attendance over 2- or 3-month periods. Therapists are tempted not to add members for fear of disrupting treatment. On occasion, the census slips, and suddenly it appears that the group will not survive without a bolus of new members. In keeping with the flexibly bound model and the characteristics of the patient population, continued longitudinal monitoring of attendance will inform the clinician of needs to add to the group roster.

DECIDING ON GROUP COMPOSITION

The chronically ill population is quite heterogeneous. Prior to beginning the recruitment process, clinicians need to define, as clearly as possible, the boundaries of group membership. Many of the principles articulated in this chapter will apply to either homogeneous or heterogeneous groups. The main emphasis, however, is in forming groups for patients exhibiting significant impairment. With varying degrees of difficulty, groups will integrate members who may be functioning at different adaptive levels, for example, a mentally retarded person with disabling impairments, or a person who more closely approximates societal role expectations. Diagnosis is of secondary importance, and patients may be included across a range of diagnostic categories. Groups composed exclusively of individuals diagnosed with schizophrenia may have difficulty interacting, and these patients may be best served through membership in a diagnostically heterogeneous group (de Bosset, 1988).

There are few specific guidelines for inclusion or exclusion for clinicians forming heterogeneous groups. A range of Axis I and Axis II diagnostic categories are associated with considerable patient impairment. It is the degree of the person's disability across social and functional realms that is a major determinant in placing a patient in a specific group.

As screening candidates progresses, clinicians tend to become protective of themselves and of the group. It is not unusual for therapists, following interviews of several candidates who are not severely impaired (i.e., relative stability, low functioning without displays of hostility, acting out, or severe thought disorganization), to exclude persons with greater disability. The opposite is also true, in that relatively higher functioning persons might not be accepted into a newly forming group in which the initial candidates appear more severely disabled. In most situations, applying such restrictions results in groups of insufficient size as well as diminished potential for stimulation provided by less obviously compatible candidates.

Patients can be included across a wide age range. We tend not to form a group with an obvious singleton, that is, a person at one or the other end of the life cycle. Groups can be limited to older individuals, including those in their 70s or 80s. Placing persons in their early 20s in such a group generally would be contraindicated. Younger, chronically ill persons can use older members as objects for identification and often benefit considerably from being with others who may be two or three decades older.

There are few reasons to exclude patients from these groups. Patients with major organic impairment or severe mental retardation should be excluded. They may be referred to homogeneous activity or social skills groups. Individuals with double diagnoses, mental illness and active substance abuse, should be referred for treatment of the substance abuse. They might be candidates for group treatment after their addiction is under control. An alternative would be a referral to a group treating both conditions simultaneously—a substance abuse and mental illness (SAMI) group. Patients in crises, usually in the form of psychotic or suicidal decompensation, should have their acceptance placed on hold until their illness has stabilized.

The course of an illness is unpredictable, and patients experiencing their initial episode of psychosis, even though they are functionally disabled at the time of assessment, generally are not good candidates for groups composed of more chronically ill patients. At an early stage of illness, when supportive resources are not well established, those persons may require more individual time and attention than a group has available. The individual's potential for recovery can be best served with a multimodal intervention that would include dyadic work.

A major reason for forming diagnostically heterogeneous groups is the practical problem of recruiting sufficient numbers of patients to begin the treatment. Often a therapist may have several patients with a particular diagnosis and wish to start a group, only to find that there are insufficient additional referrals. In most instances, the temptation to form strictly homogeneous groups should be resisted.

RECRUITING MEMBERS

Unless there is an active program in place, clinicians often overlook group treatment as a therapeutic option. This appears true even if therapists are overwhelmed by treatment requests. Thus, treating therapists perforce become ambassadors for the group modality. They often expend considerable effort networking in order to obtain sufficient referrals. As a rule of thumb, approximately 50% of those agreeing to a preparatory group interview either fail to appear for the initial screening session(s) or attend only one or two meetings following completion of that process. Therefore, 20–25 individuals may need to be contacted before a group census of 10–16 members is achieved.

Sources of patient referrals are as follows:

Therapist's own caseload
Colleagues caseload
Intake (clinic admissions)
Patient review (staff) conferences
Transfers from departing therapists
Inpatient referrals (through intake)
Continuing education seminars
Posted notice

The optimal place to recruit patients is the clinician's own dyadic caseload. Experience working individually with patients who are chronically ill provides a base for therapists to become familiar with the plethora of problems and needs facing these persons. Therapists suggesting group membership to individuals in their own caseload have the advantage of an established relationship that provides important leverage in overcoming seemingly natural reluctance to forsake the privacy of individual contact for the imagined terrors of meeting strangers and talking about oneself in a group. A number of patients will, out of compliance, rather promptly accept the clinician's recommendation for group treatment. Others will reject the suggestion outright, or they will find reasons for delay. The continuing contact with one's own patients enables clinicians to address entering a group across extended time periods. A patient's initial refusal may represent a test to determine if the therapist was serious about the benefits of group membership, and failure to follow up means that the test was not passed. Patients will agree to join if they perceive that their therapist "believes" that a group will be valuable to them, a belief that is demonstrated by the therapist's continuing but empathic exploration of patients' referrals to this treatment modality.

It is almost too obvious to point out that one of the significant advantages of coleadership, when both clinicians have individual caseloads, is that of doubling the size of the referral base. The entire recruitment and preparation process is simplified under these circumstances. Failure to recruit one's own patients suggests either incomplete knowledge about how to recruit or a previously unrecognized resistance to undertaking the enterprise. Under such circumstances, chances for success are significantly diminished.

A second referral source is the clinician's close colleagues. Informal discussion of patients among colleagues is universal, and hearing about others' problems and successes presents an opportunity to segue into discussing a possible referral for group treatment. The relationship among clinicians prevents a tendency to dismiss such suggestions out of hand. In addition, personal reminders that a search for group members is underway may stimulate colleagues to consider other patients who have been overlooked. A spin-off from this strategy is that those in the network may subsequently spread the word to others. Case managers, for example, may have clients who are not in active treatment but may benefit from referral to a group.

Linkages to the clinic intake system or to those who may be responsible for arranging the transfer of patients from departing staff members or trainees are additional important referral sources. Treatment gatekeepers significantly influence the direction of the flow of patients. The impact of having control over a clinic intake system was illustrated in the report by Yalom (1966), who, for a period of time through administrative power, was able to route all new clinic admissions to group therapy. Exclusion criteria eliminated some candidates and others refused, but Yalom successfully began nine new groups in a brief period. Most group clinicians do not exert such powerful administrative clout. By maintaining contact with an intake staff, offering consultation on perplexing patients or volunteering to conduct initial evaluations on potential group candidates, clinicians directly demonstrate their commitment to getting a group started, and they reinforce interest in finding appropriate candidates.

In most settings, therapists have opportunities to review their work with supervisors or in clinical conferences. Collaboration between the group clinicians and those in leadership positions (supervisors and conference conductors) can yield potential members. If the therapists are in such positions, they may use their authority to recommend appropriate patients for group treatment.

Patients referred from a departing clinician's caseload are potential group candidates, but they represent a risk for negative reactions. Persons subjected to the painful process of transferring from individual treatment to a group in the context of "abandonment" may respond to the departure of their therapist by retaliating against the next treatment. A negative reaction, marked by a patient's failure to complete the transfer, is more likely in the context of losing an established relationship that could ease the transition.

Another potential drawback follows from the timing of many departures in the spring or early summer. In many centers, these changes coincide with the end of a training period for some and the beginning for others. The latter clinicians are least likely to have experience with chronically ill patients and/or groups, and they may be at a disadvantage helping patients make a change in treatment modalities. Nevertheless, termination of therapists provides an opportunity to review patients' treatment and recruit group members.

A final tactic in gaining candidates is the distribution of announcements describing the group and the range of referrals desired. This is a marketing device. It alerts others to the availability of the treatment modality. Announcements are supplementary to the more personal contacts and generate occasional referrals. They serve as a useful reminder that groups are open for referrals.

Success of all recommendations for recruiting members is enhanced by a positive relationship between clinician and referral source. Educational efforts that inform clinic staff and others of the indications and detailed process of making a referral add to others' knowledge base. Inclusion of clinical vignettes counteracts relatively dry didactic material. If facilities are available, videotaped interview of a prospective group patient or of a group meeting may serve as a lively discussion stimulus. Negative responses or covert hostility on the part of others provides opportunities to correct distortions and clarify misunderstood elements in the referral process, selection procedures, or the treatment itself.

The referral form illustrated in Table 8.1 has been utilized to help remind clinicians of the essentials of a successful referral. By addressing the questions, the referring clinician helps prepare the patient for interviews with the group therapist and assists the patient in considering aspects of the treatment that will increase the likelihood of successful entry into a group.

THE INTERVIEWING PROCESS

A proposal to enter a group, whether it is accepted or rejected, stimulates patients to address relationships with others. They will respond by communicating, both consciously and unconsciously, the personal meaning of the suggestion. For some, the recommendation means that the therapist is no longer interested in them as individuals, and they are being rejected. Associations are evoked to prior experiences of loss or abandonment. A panoply of behavioral defenses may be mobilized in response to the terror of "forced" interaction with others. Patients may become overstimulated, or they may withdraw into a more schizoid or paranoid position. Whatever the patient's initial response, clinicians need to be alert to the person's communications related to the meaning of the referral. These communications can be translated, and a patient's anxieties addressed to help him or her regain inner balance.

In a system in which there is sufficient knowledge about the process of referral and in which clinicians actively support the group program, referring therapists may perform a considerable amount of the preparatory work. When patient and therapist are able to agree on the reason for the referral, and they arrive at a consensus about what problems the

TABLE 8.1. Group Therapy Referral Form

Date _____

Patient's name _____ Diagnosis _____

To (group therapist) _____

From _____

Patient's/therapist's goals for group treatment (be specific)

_____

_____

_____

1. Does the patient understand the goals?	Y N
2. Is the day and time of the group meeting compatible for the patient?	Y N
3. Are there regularly scheduled conflicts that would interfere with attendance?	Y N
4. Has the patient been in other groups (e.g., hospital, outpatient, church)?	Y N
5. Has the patient's attitudes and responses to those groups been explored?	Y N
6. Has the patient explored anxieties about joining the group?	Y N
7. Has the patient explored his or her roles usually taken in groups?	Y N
8. Do you think the patient is motivated for group treatment?	Y N

patient is going to address in the group, the entire process is simplified. Importantly, even the most highly motivated and interested individual experiences anxiety over entering a group, and referring clinicians can aid the transition by providing sufficient time to examine the patient's fears. However, such sophisticated preinterview preparation is unusual, and many individuals arrive at the group therapist's consultation room with a vague notion of what group is about, and they are present only out of compliance with the treating clinician.

In the present era of managed care, there is less motivation to prepare patients to enter a group because individual visits are not seen as cost effective. Actually, the reverse is true, because adequate preparation on the part of the referral source has the benefit of reducing time spent by the group therapist, who may expend considerable effort determining the patient's motivation and goals for joining a group.

The group clinician needs to explore with the patient in some detail the process of referral. The wide variation in preparation that patients receive prior to their arrival for pregroup interviews may result in some patients being quite reluctant to enter a group. They may have come only at the behest of their therapist, without any clear idea of why the referral was made. In addition, if the patient was being seen individually, inquiry should be made into the patient's understanding of whether he or she will continue individual sessions. The therapist should be alert to the patient's experience, either positive or negative, of the referral.

> *Example*: Anne suffered a double depression. The partially resolved major depression had been precipitated by an injury that disabled her from work, and by the death of her oldest son from AIDS. Several years before the current referral, she had considered joining a group for relatives of AIDS victims, but had not acted on the idea. Anne had only partially recovered following treatment with pharmacotherapy and individual psychotherapy, and she continued to suffer moderate depression and social isolation. She had been stimulated to consider group treatment by a sign in the clinic announcing a group for AIDS patients. Anne called her therapist, who referred her to the group therapist over the phone. In the preparatory interview, Anne recounted her symptoms at length, without mentioning group, and when the therapist began to explore her ideas about entering a group, she soon expressed reluctance to join where others would be talking about their illnesses, because that would be too upsetting. She left the session saying she wished to talk further about it with her individual therapist. Anne did not return.

There were a number of important ingredients embedded in this referral. Anne's impulsive-sounding idea for group treatment was most likely based on frustration with her dyadic treatment, and represents an enactment of those feelings. The individual therapist appeared to respond countertransferentially, by making the referral on the phone and not addressing the patient's transference. The group therapist had *not* discussed the patient with the referring clinician, and he had mistakenly assumed that Anne had discussed joining the group with her therapist. This situation is unusual, because in most instances, the referring clinician contacts the group leader to determine availability of space in the group. The irregular referral route might well have alerted the clinician to an unusual situation.

The referral also brought into focus a common dynamic—patients' anxieties evoked by listening to others' emotional problems. Yalom (1966) found that fear of emotional contagion is a reason patients may prematurely terminate. Chronically ill individuals are aware that recurrence of major symptoms is often just beyond the horizon, and they are sensitive to hearing about others' illness, because that may stimulate their own fears of decompensation and/or need for hospitalization. The fear of emotional contagion is a priority to be explored in preparing patients for group membership.

PREPARATORY TASKS

In the individual preparatory session(s), the group clinician has five tasks (Rutan & Stone, 1993):

1. Establish a preliminary alliance between patient and clinician.
2. Establish a consensus about the patient's goals.
3. Impart information about group psychotherapy.
4. Address anxieties about joining a group.
5. Inform the patient of the group agreement and gain the patient's acceptance.

Establishing Preliminary Alliances

Most chronically ill individuals suffer from major deficits in forming trusting relationships. Exploration of the process of referral and of an individual's interest in joining a group are fundamental to commencing the relationship. Some patients will present themselves with little overt reason or motivation for group therapy. They make the appointment on the recommendation of their therapist or because the doctor in the hospital said that they could benefit from a group. Their compliance hides other ideas or feelings. The clinician should not reject the patient on the basis of poor motivation, but rather he or she needs to appreciate that this posture may be adaptive for the patient who can internally limit the risks of membership by shifting responsibility to an external object. More detailed exploration of patients' prior group experiences might reveal positive and negative interactions. Some patients convey their positive feelings by displacing them on someone else who liked their group while claiming they felt negatively about it. Yet if there was not a minimum of perceived benefit, the patient might have failed the preparatory appointment.

A subgroup of patients, acting out of anxiety, put their worst foot forward. They present many obstacles to joining. In a number of instances, patients seem to be (unconsciously) testing the clinician to determine if they can manage provocations (Weiss, 1993). It is not an easy task for clinicians to differentiate between such tests and the patient's inability to directly say "no" to the referring person's offer to enter a group. Anxiety about displeasing the referring therapist or unspeakable fears about membership fuel the latter dynamic.

Other patients come to the interview having been well prepared and are able to articulate reasonable goals and ideas about groups. Nevertheless, sufficient time must be spent to demonstrate the therapist's interest in the patient as an individual and not merely as "one more member."

Because cotherapy is the most frequent group model for this population, both clinicians should attempt to develop a preliminary alliance with prospective members. Optimally, interviews should be held jointly, reflecting the leadership format. In the process of forming a new group, this can be accomplished during the time established for the meeting. Once sessions are underway, cotherapists should set aside mutually agreeable alternate times to interview prospective additions. There is a tendency when a patient has been in individual treatment with one of the group therapists to have the cotherapist conduct a private interview. The temptation should be resisted.

If times suitable to both therapists cannot be arranged, the patient then should be interviewed by each clinician separately. The least preferable model is for the interview to be conducted by only one therapist, with the plan for the patient to meet the other clinician upon entry into the group. Although patients soon find themselves attracted to one or the other clinician for a variety of reasons, meeting a cotherapist for the first time in the group skews a person's feelings in the direction of the interviewing therapist.

A treatment alliance is further enhanced as clinicians address the additional elements in the screening process. Reaching a cognitive agreement about goals, providing information about group treatment, exploring specific anxieties about entering the group, and reviewing the agreement all contribute to a positive, albeit limited, working relationship.

In interviews with patients who successfully remained in a group, several persons reflected that they had only joined to please their therapist, and had no other conscious initial motivation (McIntosh et al., 1991). However, after participating, they found that they had learned a good deal and were very pleased to have followed the therapist's recommendation.

Establishing Goals

It is the unusual chronically ill patient when contemplating entering a group who can articulate specific goals in terms of intrapsychic or interpersonal problems. It behooves the therapist then to work with the candidate to articulate reasonable goals and not reject persons who are unable to do so. If, in gathering history, helpful leads to interpersonal difficulties do not emerge, the therapist might then describe general goals that may be useful. Among these goals are learning ways of dealing with everyday problems in community living. These might range from seemingly mundane questions about shopping or arranging transportation to more complicated problems of keeping appointments or dealing with entitlement systems. It may be sufficient to accept patients who might "merely" comply with these general goals.

Patients may take therapists' acceptance of more general goals as permission to talk about disturbed interactions within their families or in their social relationships, which will lead to more precisely defined goals. For example, a patient might describe having irritably left a hospital ward meeting. Using this as a lead, other instances of action in relationships can be explored. A group goal might be to help the patient define the irritation more precisely, to identify antecedents to the feelings, or merely to find alternative behavioral solutions. By concertizing goals, patients may feel that they are collaboratively working on their problems.

Chronically ill patients rarely describe intrapsychic conflicts. Kanas (1991), working in both inpatient and outpatient settings with schizophrenic patients, articulates three goals: (1) examining and managing paranoid thinking, (2) dealing with hallucinations, and (3) exploring social relations. By addressing these tasks, the therapist gives permission to discuss what is often felt to be unspeakable and simultaneously conveys that a person's inner world may be examined. We have found that adding these elements to a general description of treatment goals, when the group is formed or when new members are added, does not evoke unmanageable anxiety in persons who do not suffer these symptoms.

There are a few goals that would exclude patients. We do not accept patients for group treatment who limit their goal to obtaining medication. These individuals, in our experience, soon become dissatisfied and terminate membership. Arrangements may be made for their treatment in a medication clinic or in a more limited medication group. Less obvious decisions for exclusion are patients with major delusional systems. Those patients presenting with rather fixed delusional systems (there are unknown persons spying or trying to hurt them, or there are sexual messages being spread about them) seem to enact a goal of convincing everyone of the veracity of their belief system. These patients become dissatisfied with the response in the group and are likely to drop from treatment. However, patients who are able to contain discussing their delusional systems and not dominate the conversation may gain considerable relief from group membership.

Example: A single woman in midlife was referred to group with the referring clinician's hopes of helping her with social isolation. She had a delusional system that chipmunks were coming from the walls and chewing on her face and nose at night, and gasses were escaping from the garage below her apartment and poisoning her food and plants. She intermittently spoke of these ideas during the first several months of her group membership. Others were skeptical of the patient's story, but were accepting of her. After several months, the patient did not mention her delusions, and although a verbally peripheral member, she continued attending until she moved from the community.

Example: A divorced man was convinced that his ex-wife was having him followed. He regaled the group with fuzzy pictures he had taken "demonstrating" cars with their headlights illuminated as proof that he was being followed. He could speak of nothing other than his complex delusional system, and attended only six meetings before stopping without notice.

Imparting Information

Prospective members should be provided with basic information about group treatment. A balance needs to be struck between a too detailed description that evokes anxiety and insufficient information that leaves candidates uninformed. The therapist tells patients of the time, place, size of the group, and, with the flexibly bound model, the usual number of patients in attendance. Patients can be told in advance that the therapist does not introduce topics, but members may talk about whatever they choose.

An important informational element is that the therapist may have contact with the patient's other care providers. It is essential that permission be obtained to maintain contact with mental health clinicians, case managers, general medical caregivers, or appropriate agencies. An occasional person may be hesitant about giving permission for these contacts. In most instances, following the opportunity to discuss their concerns and an explanation that collaboration among service providers will enhance their care, patients will give permission. If the reluctance persists, then the clinicians may chose to delay admission or still accept that patient, recognizing the limitations inherent in being unable to collaborate with other caregivers.

Because many patients referred for group treatment are receiving medication, they may wonder if that component of their treatment will take place in the group. How medications will be provided should be clarified in advance in order to allay anxiety and assure individuals that the medication component of their treatment will receive attention.

Dealing with Anticipatory Anxiety

Patients exhibit a wide range of overt anxiety as they contemplate entering a group. A proportion of the chronic population shows no evidence of overt concern about meeting strangers. They appear to join a group without asking many questions or displaying feelings. Some patients wall off their entire experience of psychosis (McGlashan et al., 1975), and it may be that others will do the same in preparing themselves for a novel interpersonal experience. Like any other aspect of their lives, patients protect themselves against anxiety-laden experiences. The ordinary human experience is such that this behavior appears odd, and the clinician is tempted to challenge the "denial." Therapists may acknowledge the temptation to themselves, but the patient's emotional position should be empathically explored rather than confronted.

Some patients can acknowledge their anxieties. The fears of emotional contagion and hearing about others' illnesses can be alleviated by reviewing patients' hospital experiences, where they have been in contact with more acutely disturbed individuals. Nevertheless, the task of meeting strangers is anxiety evoking, and for many patients may seem monumental. Here a strategy of rehearsal can be useful. In addition to exploring prior experiences in meeting new people (church, school, family events), patients can be instructed to role play in the preparatory interviews. The patients' sense of having prepared serves to lessen their anxiety.

Some patients cannot directly address their anxieties and yet they communicate their feelings in metaphor or displacement. Although it is unusual, some individuals will present their anxieties by reporting a dream that is not necessarily of recent origin. The dream may express general anxiety or more direct interpersonal concerns. By attending to the process of patients' associations to the question of concerns about entering a group, clinicians can translate these metaphors and address the feelings more directly. In this manner, therapists also convey to patients how they will be listening and responding in the group.

The Therapeutic Agreement

The framework for the therapeutic process is contained in the agreement reached between patient and therapist. The agreement provides information to the patient and the clinician alike. It is an attempt to create a balance between providing sufficient structure to contain the treatment enterprise and minimizing an authoritarian structure (Rutan & Stone, 1993).

The agreement delimits place, frequency, time, and duration of the treatment, and as such creates a boundary between the group and the external world. The agreement also attempts to provide guidelines about the relationship between information exchanged across the external boundary, that is, what information from outside may be brought into the meetings and what taking place in the session may be taken outside. In addition, the agreement defines appropriate behaviors that are to take place within the meeting and more specifically addresses the relationships among the members and with the therapist (the internal boundary).

The agreement should be presented in the preparatory interviews. The information, although seemingly straightforward, is actually quite dense and is not readily absorbed. Sufficient time should be allowed for the patient to discuss the elements of the agreement. Some clinicians provide a written copy in order to reinforce what has been presented verbally. The agreement is repeated when a new group is begun, and when new members join an ongoing group.

The elements of the agreement include the following:

Attendance expectations. In traditional outpatient groups, patients are expected to attend each session on time and remain throughout the meeting. In the flexibly bound model, this expectation is modified, and a patient is asked to attend four consecutive meetings and then determine with the therapist(s) how frequently, ranging from weekly to monthly, he or she will attend (McIntosh et al., 1991). This negotiation is conducted at the end of a meeting, in the presence of others. Patients are asked to announce in the group any forthcoming absences, and they are asked to notify the therapist (or the clinic) if they are unable to attend a meeting.

Therapists also inform members when they will be absent or if there is to be an interruption in the meeting schedule (vacations or holidays). In addition, when new members are to be introduced, the group will be notified in advance—no new child will be brought into the family unannounced. This portion of the agreement contributes in a major way in establishing an external group boundary.

Members agree to work toward their goals. This portion of the agreement serves primarily as a reminder that patients have discussed goals. In presenting the agreement in the group, the clinician might briefly outline the different goals that have been agreed upon without identifying specific individuals: "The goals that we have talked about include trying to improve relationships with our family or with others; to find ways of making our lives more comfortable; to exchange ideas about the impact of being ill upon our relationships; or to discuss problems with medications." In some instances, specific symptoms of major illness might be included, such as managing responses to hallucinations, clarifying problems in thinking, or overcoming feelings of depression. By articulating these latter goals, the therapist "normalizes" them and gives patients permission to openly discuss them.

These goals are sufficiently general to include many of the patients' issues. It is unusual for patients to articulate wishes to work on strong feelings, particularly anger. Some might wish to find ways of overcoming their shyness or anxiety in meeting and talking with others. Patients manage these latter affects more readily, and in the initial group phases, examining those feelings does not derail the group as does examining angry affects. This portion of the agreement contributes to establishment of an internal boundary.

Members agree to put their feelings into words, not actions. Members are relieved when the agreement includes a clear statement regarding abstinence from physical violence. Other forms of action, however, are accepted and seldom commented upon by the therapist, although the timing of those behaviors provides information about the manner in which each person may handle relationships. Some patients have difficulty remaining in their seats for the full meeting, and they may pace during the session. Other settings provide coffee, and patients may leave the circle to get a cup during a period of personal or group tension. Clinical judgment is required to determine if such behaviors should be directly addressed, or if they should be accepted as communication about patients' inner states, not necessitating comment.

Example: Betty, a single, mildly mentally retarded woman, spoke with a high-pitched voice that had little modulation. Shortly after entering a meeting, Betty began to demonstrate the effects of a recent leg injury by limping about the room, and at the same time loudly attempting to explain her injury. The discomfort generated in the room was manifested by others shifting in their chairs and averting their eyes. The therapist, after a very brief interval, firmly asked Betty to return to her seat. She protested but was able to tolerate the limits. The patients' associations were to experiences in which others were out of control. The cotherapists proceeded to assist Betty in explaining that she felt she was unable to describe her injury and had to demonstrate it. Members were encouraged to describe their discomfort and their thoughts, which included ideas that they would not return the following week. By the end of the session, all had agreed to come back.

Patients also act verbally. A direct critical or hostile attack by one member against another is a violation of this element in the agreement. Members' sense of safety rapidly diminishes in situations in which patients are allowed to "express their feelings" through verbal attacks on one another. Clinicians may choose to try to understand the precipitant for such attacks and interpret the sequence within the general framework of the attack being a response to narcissistic injury (Stone, 1993a). This may not be successful, and the therapist may need to set firm limits on verbal attacks, indicating that members may talk about their own feelings but not attack others. If this is ineffective, the offending patient may be asked to leave the session until he or she regains control (see Chapter 13).

Extragroup contacts. In contrast to groups composed primarily of higher functioning individuals, minimal emphasis is placed upon this element of the agreement. Likewise, personal anonymity is not maintained to the same degree. Members quickly share last names, where they live, and phone numbers. They often have common acquaintances living in the same neighborhood or attending the same church. Indeed, members may have considerable contact with one another outside the sessions. It is not unusual for telephone networks to become established in which members are in frequent contact with one another. These contacts are often viewed as very helpful during periods when a person is stressed. Not uncommonly, one person will bring information to the group about the reason for another person's missing a meeting, information that had not been previously provided to the therapist.

Members ride the bus together and become involved in friendships outside the session. One phobic woman had been brought to the sessions by her family. As she improved, she was able to arrange to meet another member after only a short ride alone on the bus, and they completed the trip to the clinic together.

Not surprisingly some patients are excluded from the extragroup networks and may experience negative effects from their feelings of exclusion. Some individuals may "abuse" others with frequent phone calls.

> *Example*: A schizophrenic woman would call others in the group well after midnight when she either could not sleep or was overtly upset about an event during the day. It was only after several months that this came to light in the group. The patient was instructed to stop making the calls and contact the 24-hour psychiatric emergency service instead.

Eventually, most outside contacts that create difficulty will be brought into the group. The concept that outside contacts are meaningful in understanding members' internal and interpersonal world is difficult to convey. Thus a comment will suffice that if outside contacts are important, then members can bring that up in the group.

Therapists should maintain a neutral attitude regarding outside contacts among members. Some clinicians encourage or even require patients to socialize or to actively intervene in circumstances when a member is experiencing some sort of need for help. Patients suffer a good deal in their relationship to those in authority, and clinicians should be very wary of imposing requirements or making suggestions, with the exception of those activities that become destructive to the group process, in regard to how members behave toward one another.

Agreement about fees. Patients are asked to be responsible for their fees. In most settings, patients are supported by public funds and the payment is made to the clinic for the services provided. Patients themselves pay either no fee or a minimal fee. What is required is that patients cooperate with the clinic to ensure that forms are completed. Englander (1989) found that clinicians' ratings of group cohesion were positively correlated with explicit discussion of fees as an element in the group agreement. This finding held both in private practice and in clinics where fees were not paid to the clinician. This component of the agreement provides patients with a sector of their treatment in which they can act responsibly. There are very few persons who are completely comfortable accepting free care. By responsibly completing forms, patients demonstrate their cooperation and commitment to treatment.

Maintaining confidentiality of the members. This element of the agreement is presented last because it is necessary to emphasize its importance. Much of what is said in presenting the agreement will be misunderstood, misinterpreted, or forgotten. By making this the final piece of the agreement, the clinician can gain patients' attention and reinforce the significance of confidentiality for the treatment. Patients will discuss their group experiences with others, and this should not be discouraged. Rather, the therapist should indicate that in order for the group to function effectively, patients need to feel safe and that what they say will be kept confidential. This point can be elaborated by explaining that in discussing a meeting with nonmembers, identities of those present in the group are not to be revealed. In most instances, this component will be respected.

Agreement transgressions (boundary crossings and violations) are inevitable and provide considerable information about members' relationships to one another, with the therapist, or with their image of the group as a whole. The therapist must differentiate between relatively benign or even therapeutically useful crossings and those that are group destructive. Some distinctions are easy to make. Other violations, which at first seem to be benign, may have a dark side. The distinctions often emerge in the treatment context and may be initially expressed in metaphorical communication. Clear limits are necessary to protect individual and group functioning.

SUMMARY

In this chapter, the practical elements of deciding on group organization, composition, recruitment, interviewing processes, and the preparatory tasks have been addressed. These elements may be time consuming and often are not considered essential. Failure by clinicians to responsibly attend to these aspects, however, may turn a potentially successful group program into one hovering on extinction.

The final section in this chapter examined the group agreement, which is an essential element in creating a safe therapeutic environment. The flexibly bound model represents one modification of the traditional arrangements.

NINE

THE ROLE OF THE THERAPIST

*I believe that trainees should learn to think about their
work and not just about their patients. And the main
thing about their work that they should think about is
the problem they have with it.*

—FRIEDMAN (1988, p. 540)

The role of the therapist is central in developing an effective therapeutic enterprise. In a group of seriously and persistently ill patients,
it is all the more important because of the therapist's necessary role
functions. The task may be daunting and time consuming. The
model of a therapist quietly engaged in analyzing intrapsychic conflicts is
insufficient to encompass the task. For instance, the clinician must work
collaboratively with colleagues who assist patients who receive necessary
services such as housing, transportation, and other medical care (Stone,
1991). At other times, the therapist may meet with family members or
assist in the involuntary hospitalization of an acutely decompensated
group member.

In assuming therapeutic responsibilities for a group, clinicians must
attend to their own needs as well as those of the patients. Being aware of
aspects of one's own motivations enables therapists to more readily track
the treatment process. The major tasks undertaken in helping patients then
can be more readily addressed.

THERAPISTS' CHARACTERISTICS AND MOTIVATIONS

Certain personal characteristics enhance clinicians' potential for success.
In addition to a willingness to collaborate with other professionals,

therapists must exhibit a capacity to tolerate and contain intense unspoken and unconscious conflicts, to be able to maintain a balance between activity and inactivity, to respect a slow rate of change, and to gain personal satisfaction from seemingly small change. Chronically ill patients, almost by definition, have extended experiences of failed interpersonal relationships. They cautiously enter into new relationships, burdened by their prior experiences, and only slowly and in small increments do they allow others into their inner world. Change may be subtle and manifest itself in the tone of one member's inquiry of another or in the timing or content of a question. Even though a comment may not be in order, the clinician needs to note these changes in the group transactions.

Therapists must bear and contain intense affects that members cannot easily examine or tolerate in themselves. In particular, patients avoid and project feelings of anger and rage into the therapist. But other feelings are difficult for patients to handle as well, and clinicians may find themselves bored, envious, disinterested, or experiencing seemingly unrelated fantasies about their own lives. Therapists' disappointments with patients' real accomplishments are frequent: when a group member finds part-time employment only to be fired within a very short period, when a member continues to be abused by a spouse or a casual friend, when a person fails to be assertive in a seemingly simple situation. Keeping one's balance and therapeutic investment is a challenge for all clinicians, but particularly so in working with this population, because of the many levels of difficulties encountered.

Among the familiar elements that serve as barriers for therapists' involvement are patients' limited collaboration in the sick role, their tenuous capacity to make emotional contact, their slow rate of change, and their needs for multiple services.

Therapists' needs, in part fueling their entry into the field, require attention in order to help maintain their optimal functioning. Friedman (1988) examined clinicians' motivations and actions (including thoughts) that are at work in the therapist-in-action. He enumerated three motives for clinicians' actions, independent of their theoretical orientation, that served to help them maintain their balance: (1) to act like a therapist, (2) to satisfy curiosity, and (3) to elicit something desirable. Recognizing these attributes is primarily for the benefit of the therapist. However, they may also be of value to patients, who will be rewarded by their clinicians' cognizance of the many elements contributing to the treatment relationship.

To Act Like a Therapist

Embedded in a therapist's theoretical orientation are plans that will propel treatment toward its goals. Dynamically trained clinicians value free associations and generally discourage behavioral actions as they work toward helping patients gain greater self-understanding. Thus when clinicians are perplexed, they may employ tactics that will encourage verbalization, such as asking questions or remaining silent in hope of stimulating discussion. These are actions that fit into a treatment plan and help clinicians continue to feel as if they are behaving within the ideal of a dynamically trained therapist.

As with any set of rules for behavior, techniques employed by the clinician may fall flat, particularly if they are applied in rote fashion. Extended silences may at times stimulate patients to focus on their inner thoughts and feelings, whereas, another time, it may be most important to keep them connected to their interpersonal world and not encourage deep introspection. Inquiries made in a routine fashion or employed too frequently may be experienced by members as stereotyped and unempathic. The neophyte's question "What are you feeling?" may encourage members' self-examination, but used too frequently or routinely will have a counterproductive impact.

Members may comment to the clinician, "I knew you would say that," or "You always ask that question." These remarks may be a commentary about the therapist's stereotyped responses, or they may be a communication about the patient's sense of consistency and reliability that has reassuring qualities. Such comments require the therapist's self scrutiny and exploration with the patient, but they may reflect a slavish adherence to a theoretical stance or a diminution of curiosity.

To Satisfy Curiosity

Therapists are fundamentally curious about human behavior. They want to know why people behave in particular ways, or what they can do to modify behaviors. Theory influences curiosity. For instance, the dynamic therapist examines defenses, drives, adaptional modes, and personality structures. The behavioral therapist may attempt to formulate a hierarchy of fears to help a patient overcome a phobia. Theory may be organizing for therapists in helping them to understand behavior and to point the way to further inquiry, but it may also be constricting. Clinicians in pursuit of confirming theory may have their curiosity constrained and may ignore data that do not fit.

Curiosity may be focused on patients' here-and-now interactions, on the developmental basis for the feelings or behaviors, or on future implications for what has transpired. The clinician's interest may be stimulated by hearing a patient's story as illuminating the reality of an event or as a metaphor for the therapeutic encounter. Slavish adherence to a single theoretical position, which supports the clinician's acting like a therapist, will diminish curiosity.

Therapists need to develop a curiosity about their own countertransferential responses to the therapeutic interactions. Feelings of frustration, boredom, sadness, tenderness, or anger all may be reflections of unexpressed emotions within the group. Seemingly intrusive memories of one's own experience may be a source of considerable information about unexpressed feelings conveyed in the patient–therapist interactions. Clinicians' capacities to monitor and utilize those countertransferences will enhance their therapeutic effectiveness as well as satisfy their curiosity. For example, a therapist might find him- or herself thinking about a summer vacation during a meeting. This might be an expression of a wish to leave the treatment because of intense unexpressed negative affects, or it might be a container of an equally troublesome problem in expressing warm, positive feelings.

Therapists achieve considerable inner satisfaction when their curiosity is satisfied. There are generally sufficient data to satisfy if clinicians can learn to ask themselves the proper questions. They may explore their own inner responses, members' behaviors, or the state of the group functioning.

Some questions may be asked, only to be met with a "non response." These transactions optimally should stimulate curiosity rather than stultify it. Many questions will only remain as part of the inner processes examined by the clinician.

To Elicit Something Desirable

Therapists search for something beyond satisfaction of their intellectual curiosity. Friedman (1988) states, "The therapist's undeliberate search for interactive response plays a special role in psychotherapy" (p. 107). The therapist is seeking an interaction. This is not necessarily verbal but may be transmitted along nonverbal channels that often are explained as "energy."

> *Example*: The concept is illustrated in a quote from Garry Kasparov, a world-class chess champion engaged in a match against a computer: "When playing versus a human being there's energy going between us. Today I was puzzled because I felt no energy—kind of like a black hole into which my energy could disappear. But I discovered a new source of energy, from the audience to me, and I thank you very much for this enormous energy supply" (cited in Leithauser, 1990, p. 65).

Certainly, the analogy comparing chronically ill patients with computerized chess is slightly overdrawn, but in the extreme, some patients have dehumanized themselves, as exemplified by one individual who conceives of himself as a "fax robot."

Chronically ill patients erect barriers to emotional involvement, and treatment may potentially proceed in a deadening fashion. The barriers may come in the familiar form of schizoid type presentations, but they may also appear in overly clinging or demanding relationships in which the clinician's experience is that of a function, rather than a collaborative person. Transactions then are experienced, described in self psychology as one of a self–selfobject transference.

In groups, the therapist's experience is often expressed silently as wondering, "Why can't they relate to one another?"

Conversely, patients interacting in unexpected and sensitively human ways may be very gratifying. A central component of the good therapeutic session is not merely confirmation of one's theory, but contains genuine interaction among the members or with the clinician.

> *Example*: Illustrative of such interaction was the "breakthrough" exhibited by a very passive, dependent man, who assertively told a dominating woman with schizoaffective disorder that she had interrupted him. The woman, who was only slowly modifying her behavior, surprisingly apologized and turned to listen. Several other members then remarked on the man's "sticking up for himself." Almost all the members participated in this socially ordinary-appearing interaction. Indeed it was the ordinariness of the exchanges, representing a changed atmosphere, that was the "something desirable."

Therapists need to be tolerant of their inner responses. Accepting and being able to sort through often disturbing affects can help clinicians determine what is aroused in them by the patients who in turn may have evoked their own unresolved conflicts. Those experiences and memories can be used as a channel of communication from the patient or the group, which in turn can be explored with the members. This use of countertransferences (the therapist's affects) must be scrutinized as carefully as possible to prevent the clinician from responding primarily out of his or her own unresolved conflicts.

Feelings aroused often evoke fears in therapists that they are as "sick" as their patients. Clinicians' anxieties about merging with the group or specific members can interfere with their capacity to use themselves as therapeutic instruments. It may be useful to appreciate that most of the ways patients express themselves can be found in the depths of everyone's inner world, and the therapist does well *not* to assume the emotional stance, "that's not me."

THERAPISTS' TASKS

In the formally designated time for group sessions, therapists may conceptualize their task as creating an atmosphere in which patients can develop sufficient trust (which may be an achievement in itself) to expose and work with their fundamental interpersonal and intrapsychic disturbances. For heuristic purposes, these tasks may be examined as seven separate elements (Stone, 1993a):

1. Managing boundaries
2. Bonding members
3. Identifying themes
4. Managing affect
5. Handling metaphors
6. Promoting problem solving
7. Promoting self-understanding (insight)

Managing Boundaries

In order for the group to become a useful therapeutic experience, patients need to develop a sense of safety, which might be considered akin to the safety required by a small child who begins exploring the world. In group treatment, the important boundaries are those that contain the group, defining what is inside and what is outside, and those separating members from one another and from the therapist. The group agreement (see Chapter 8) is an initial step in helping define boundaries. Firm but penetrable boundaries for the group and the members, however, evolve during the therapeutic process. They are a product of the therapist's abilities and the members' capacities, which are significant developmental achievements, to open themselves sufficiently to allow input without fearing dissolution and, as well, the ability to reconstitute themselves following penetration.

The external group boundary defines who is in the group and who is not, and includes the time, duration, place, and type of information to be brought into the treatment setting. These boundaries are variably permeable. Being too rigid or too porous will interfere with treatment (Rice & Rutan, 1987).

The therapist selects individuals who will cross the external boundary and enter into group membership. In working with chronically mentally ill individuals, membership is not always as distinct as it is with higher functioning groups.

A characteristic of many groups is intermittent attendance. As described in the formation of a group with flexible boundaries (Chapter 8), not all members attend weekly, and groups form with core and peripheral subgroups. An additional consideration arises when a patient, who has disappeared from treatment, and who no longer remains on the clinic roll, suddenly appears for a group session. A boundary may be crossed, and the therapist must decide whether the individual may be allowed to remain or be asked to leave. Such a decision is part of the human judgment exercised by the therapist (Singer et al., 1975). Therapeutic implications flow from either decision. Klein (1992) describes the impact of a hyperactive former member's intrusion upon a group and the subsequent discussion following the person's departure as leading to a productive discussion of patients' emotional dilemmas of "safety" achieved by maintaining tight personal boundaries and the price of loneliness concomitant with those behaviors.

Group boundary crossings may result from the limited social network of many chronically ill individuals. If the clinic does not provide for care of small children, caregiver patients are faced with the dilemma of either not attending or bringing children to the group. A prohibition against including children in a meeting may limit patients' options. Some groups tolerate and can utilize the presence of young children, particularly if the room is of sufficient size to allow children a degree of activity. Information about parenting or grandparenting capacities may become more available when interactions with children are directly observable (Stone, 1983). Not all groups are structured in a manner that accepts children, but for those that do, their inclusion in a session provides an opportunity to examine another sector of patients' interactive capacities.

Another consequence of patients' diminished social networks is their propensity to transport relationships formed in the group into their external support systems. Extending relationships from the group to the external world may be growth promoting for an isolated individual, but the response among members may be destructive to the treatment process because unmanageable affects, including envy, jealousy, and feelings of exclusion or competitiveness, are aroused. Therapists face a considerable dilemma in determining the management of such situations. In general, it is counterproductive to criticize or prohibit such meetings.

A somewhat different situation arises when a member is ill or in the hospital and others express a wish to call or visit. Should the therapist reveal the nature of the illness or provide a phone number or the name of the hospital? What boundaries should be maintained even if the ill person requests that the therapist invite members to visit? No guidelines will save the therapist from some uncertainty.

Crucial to creating a group environment is closing the door, which is a concrete representation of the boundary. A therapist may not wish to offend tardy members, and consequently will delay closing the door. Similarly, members arriving late may leave the door open, signaling that others, arriving even later, may be expected, or the act may represent a denial of their own lateness. The therapist needs to close the door or ask the latecomer to close it. Little, if any, therapeutic work can be accomplished with an open door.

One strategy that protects the external boundary is provision of coffee in the treatment room. When tension rises, patients can then leave the circle, pour coffee, and still remain in the room. Eventually, as members can handle such tension, those actions diminish, or they may be explored when a sufficient treatment alliance has been established.

The internal boundary defines relationships among members. Elements of the agreement directly address the nature and content of members' interactions with each other and with the therapist. An instruction that encourages discussion of hallucinations, delusions, and paranoid thinking gives permission to address topics that are often avoided (Kanas, 1985). Similarly, the therapist's comment that any announcements will be made at the beginning of the session and that his or her planned absences will be announced in advance sets a tone of respect and a beginning security that no surprises will be sprung after the opening minutes.

Members' work is defined as trying to put ideas and feelings into words and not into action. The emphasis on verbal exchange creates a physical space and begins to set an atmosphere for verbal space. Therapists need to protect members against verbal as well as physical aggression. Dynamic processes such as offering up a member to determine the quality of safety or the process of scapegoating are examples of emotional transactions that penetrate others' boundaries. Failure to attend to these boundary crossings may lead to a scapegoated victim departing from the group.

An exception to the guideline of putting feelings into words is established by the presence of a coffee pot in the group room. Here patients do act to relieve tension, and the behavior may become a norm that is difficult to alter but may remain a useful alternative to more directly expressing feelings.

Example: Members managed the tension they experienced following the addition of a monopolizing hypomanic woman by more frequently refilling their cups. When the newcomer became more integrated into the group, in substantial part due to the positively tinged feelings among members, the trips diminished. The coffee allowed a certain splitting to occur, and negative feelings were "metabolized" into more manageable affects.

Example: A woman diagnosed with schizoaffective disorder, in anticipation of the group being subjected to a visitor, brought a home-baked cake to the group. Members and therapist partook and commented admiringly on her baking ability. The patient responded by purchasing equipment to further decorate her baking and thereby stopped borrowing the same materials from her mother. However, later, when she had missed a series of sessions in response to group tension, she produced another cake, which was clearly a peace offering. In this instance, the feelings around the absences were addressed to the extent that seemed possible.

The essence of treatment is in the interaction among patients. The external boundary provides the frame, and the internal boundary helps define the quality and nature of members' relationships.

Bonding Members

Bonding with the group is initiated in the preparatory interviews with the therapist. This accounts for some of the apparent dependency behavior patients exhibit. The therapist then makes active efforts to bond individuals to subgroups (Agazarian & Janoff, 1993) or to the group as whole. Individuals' propensities to fulfill certain roles (e.g., scapegoat, spokesperson, identified patient) serve to isolate and inhibit flexibility. By the therapist's actively linking individuals, they are no longer alone. In the group developmental schema, bonding promotes movement from pregroup or parallel processes in the entry phase to a more connected interactive phase.

Each person enters his or her group as a singleton. The very process of gaining a sense of belonging to a group and having satisfactory relationships becomes a participant's goal. Some individuals will bring to the fore their social skills by beginning with small talk. Questions such as "Where do you live?," "Where do you work?," and "Do you have children?" are opening stages in trying to determine how and in what areas one can link with another.

Upon entering a group, the limited social skills of many chronically ill persons emerge in stark relief to those who are more skilled. Their curiosity about others appears minimal, and much attention, if expressed, is toward the therapist. Small-talk equivalents are inquiries about medications or dates and places of hospital treatment. Many therapists incorrectly hear patients' discussions of medication as a concrete request or as a metaphor for unmet oral dependency needs, and overlook the bonding that takes place as members exchange information about psychotropic drugs or medical illness.

Bonding can be effected in sectors of affect ("The two of you were feeling hurt and ignored, Ms. A, when your children ignored your birthday, and, Mr. B, when your friend did not invite you to go fishing"), in similarities of experiences ("Both of you lived with your grandmother after you left your home in the country"), or in ideas ("You both hope that your children will be more attentive to you").

Additional bonding takes place outside of the group. Patients who are frightened of the relatively unstructured group environment will seek commonalities or linkages with others in situations they believe to be more manageable. This may begin at the clinic registration desk, in the waiting room, on the way home, or through nascent phone networks. Subgroups may bond, but they also may split off conflicts and make them unavailable for discussion. Therapeutic judgment is required to properly time interventions that address the limiting aspects of outside subgroups while not undermining their positive aspects.

Individuals often split their feelings and experiences, and through developing functional subgroups, patients are better positioned to explore conflict.

> *Example*: Mr. C, annoyed with being honked at while waiting in his car at a busy intersection, expressed his displeasure by giving the "finger" to the other driver. He was startled and frightened when, at the next light, the driver got out of his car and started pounding on Mr. C's car windows. Hearing this story, the members spontaneously subgrouped. One member told Mr. C to contain his feelings, and another member joined this subgroup by telling him that his anger must have come from the past and was out of place. A third person commented that he had behaved like Mr. C on a number of occasions and felt better for doing it. This subgrouping then enabled members to explore their differences without feeling alone.

A more difficult task is engaging all patients with a sense of belonging to the entire group. Group-as-a-whole interventions cannot address the nuances of each person's participation in the process, and as a result can potentially be injurious. With that reservation in mind, nevertheless, whole-group interpretations help link the members with the treatment endeavor and increase a sense of a shared experience. Silent individuals may then be drawn into the conversation if the intervention strikes a positive note. If differences with the comment emerge, then an opportunity is presented to promote subgrouping and avoid producing singletons.

When confronted with conflicts with authority, patients often will recruit silent members to increase group solidarity before they risk expressing criticism or anger. This process often takes place in the context of a change in the boundary (a difficult new member, or an interruption in the regular meeting schedule) and may be initially expressed in a displacement. The infrequent expression of anger toward the therapist is most often preceded by recruitment activity.

Developing a patient's capacity to act entirely independently is generally an unrealistic goal. Many are dependent upon public funds for their subsistence. Sharing frustrations and victories with the "system" bonds members and points them in the direction of more adaptive solutions to old conflicts.

Identifying Themes

Bonding processes are enhanced when a common theme is identified in patients' associations. To find overt or covert commonalities may require considerable integration by the clinician. A theme may emerge in a single session or may become manifest over many weeks or months, particularly when the salience is high.

Certain themes are worked on in many different ways. Among the more frequently addressed issues are isolation, loneliness, and aloneness. Members express concerns about the impact of their illness upon them, their prognoses, the treatment they are receiving, their relationships within and outside the family, and the acceptance of mental illness by others. Other themes deal with shame over their illness, boundaries of sex and aggression, trust–distrust, and acceptance.

Issues may be stimulated by a member's association or by interactions within the group. Responses may range from direct expression of the theme to defenses against associated affects.

> *Example*: In one group, Ms. D, who had a long-standing hostile/dependent relationship with her well-to-do sister, bemoaned her situation of having to depend on others to take her to the grocery, and she ruminated about moving to an apartment more convenient to the store. Two members talked about how they took care of others, and whenever they asked for a favor it was refused or only done with a grumpy countenance. Another member, who also sacrificed herself excessively, complained that only two people in her apartment complex offered to help after her heart attack, when she was unable to shop for herself. They talked about how they could not depend on people, but how it was necessary in order to survive.

The therapist could not identify any recent group stress that had precipitated these associations. The theme involved members' anxieties over wishes to be cared for and the failure of their solutions of obsessively caring for others in hopes of assuring reciprocity. The limited real resources of this population stimulate many similar themes that may be addressed in the external situation. Nevertheless, therapists need to carefully search for stimuli for such associations within the group transferences.

Improvement and beginning exploration of entering the work force stimulate in patients a spectrum of themes addressing whether their illness should be revealed, the public's attitude toward their illness—and of course, covertly, what the clinician "really thinks of them," or even more personally, their own thoughts about their illness. Will the stress of work make them ill, or what might happen to their disability payments if they do succeed?

Themes may be explored from a variety of perspectives that enable patients to subgroup and proceed with exploring differences in a therapeutically useful fashion. Talking about work can bring into focus numerous issues that can be elaborated into themes. As in the prior example, patients may explore consequences of revealing to employers that they are ill, or they may choose to withhold such information and explore the implications of that action. The therapist must balance allowing themes to develop and risk a lack of focus against the possibility of prematurely intervening and interfering with the emergence of an important issue.

Managing Affect

Affects are conceptualized as "organized and organizing aspects of mental functioning" (Shapiro & Emde, 1992, p. x). They may be examined from biological, developmental, and social perspectives. The disability of many chronically ill individuals is increased as a result of deficits in identifying, labeling, and tolerating affects. Expression of and defenses against emotions are of major clinical importance, and the group setting provides an *in vivo* opportunity to study these processes.

Emotional states are conveyed through verbal and nonverbal channels. The latter are expressed through physical activity, body attitudes, facial expression, or in the tone, rate, or volume of speech. The potential for unspoken affects to spread with lightning speed (emotional contagion) through the group is considerable, and therapists are not immune to the spread of feelings as they find themselves filled with the same feelings as the members. Indeed, the clinician's awareness and ability to use his or her feelings (countertransferences) are vital in understanding communications within the treatment setting.

Members' capacities to tolerate and manage feelings contribute greatly to group dynamics. Themes may be derailed and norms established based on an individual's capacity, in collusion with others, to tolerate feelings. Nonresponse to an affect-laden communication is a simple but often effective extinguisher of emotional expression. Norms, often not conscious, develop that restrain investigation of feelings.

Group development may hinge on members' perceptions of emotional safety. One "strategy," not consciously planned, is to put forth a member who personifies the issues in the preconscious hope that a problem will be resolved. Members may encourage one person to behave in a manner that will test the situation, for example, criticizing the therapist, trying to obtain special attention, or indicating that the therapy is not useful. The underlying message involves determination of what is safe. Patients' unacceptable or negative feelings are often managed by placing them in vulnerable members who serve as scapegoats. In this process, members rid themselves of the "unacceptable" feelings but in the process become diminished, because the projected feelings are not available for exploration. The therapist's task is to help members "own" their projections, thereby achieving greater affect integration and simultaneously relieving the scapegoat of an extra affective burden (Agazarian & Janoff, 1993). Achieving this goal is frequently impossible without extended periods of treatment.

Of particular salience is members' capacities to tolerate separations, which occur with much greater frequency in group than in dyadic treatment. Diminished attendance before and after therapists' vacations or interruptions caused by a clinic holiday is common. Patients may respond to a forthcoming treatment interruption across several channels. They respond with bodily expression, in the tone or rate of their speech, or through metaphors of authority figures failing to fulfill their responsibilities.

> *Example*: In one group, following announcement of an interruption due to the therapist's planned absence, a member insistently questioned the therapist about where he was going, suggesting several likely vacation spots. With some hesitation, the clinician responded that he would be away for a Jewish holiday. The patient then commented that he understood, because his individual therapist also would be away for several days for the same reason. The group continued to work, and there seemed no reference to the interruption until several minutes prior to end of the meeting, when the patient associated to his disappointment that a friend had canceled a recent golf game. The patient rejected an alternate offer and then neglected to call his friend the next day as agreed.

The "passive–aggressive" reaction to his friend expresses the patient's anger at the therapist's forthcoming departure. The message was delivered at the end of the meeting in order to minimize the risk, in the patient's fantasy, that his communication would evoke retaliation.

The therapist's tasks include helping individuals identify feelings.

Patients appear to suffer alexithymia and seem unable to label feelings (Swiller, 1988). They may suffer with somatic symptoms that are characteristic of either regression or developmental arrest. Translation of these symptoms into identifiable emotions begins the process of helping patients label their emotional responses (Krystal, 1974).

Many individuals are familiar with hurt and angry feelings. Anger is often difficult to manage, particularly when there is a threat to act. On occasion, anger bubbles over either into yelling or into threats of violence. In those circumstances, patients need to be firmly and clearly reminded that they cannot act on their feelings, which would include shouting at one another. If such an admonition is ignored, members may be firmly asked to leave until they regain control of their feelings.

> *Example*: During one session, a patient with major character pathology refused to stop verbally abusing another member or to comply with the request to leave. The therapist, not knowing what to do, left the room, looking for help, and returned with a very large case manager who sat in the circle. This show of force quieted the patient, who over an extended period of time was able to reflect on the precipitant for this outburst. No group work can be accomplished when there is a threat to physical safety.

Patients are reassured if the therapist or group serves as an appropriate container for anger. However, the research on expressed emotion has demonstrated that schizophrenic patients are vulnerable to an exacerbation of their illness in an atmosphere of high levels of anger. Depressed individuals also are sensitive to relapse in the context of angry expressions, which they may interpret as a threat to the relationship (Hooley et al., 1986). Kanas (1985) has demonstrated the counterproductive aspects of encouraging or allowing expression of angry feelings in time-limited groups composed of schizophrenic patients. The inexact equation of a group and a family, however, does appear salient to patients' capacities to manage anger.

Therapists often can interrupt angry outbursts by attending to the treatment process and searching for a precipitant for their expressions. A seemingly innocuous narcissistic injury may be experienced as disruptive to a vulnerable patient who then responds with anger. Patients can address feelings of loss, disappointment, or hurt much more readily than they can those of anger.

> *Example*: For several years a man and woman had carried on a continuing battle that had not been easily amenable to containment. The therapist noted that the two antagonists seemed to be talking amiably as she entered the room. The woman, who suffered from

schizophrenia, turned to the therapist to ask several questions, at which point the man began berating her. The therapist commented on the sequence, and for the first time the man said that he had been hurt by the woman's turning her attention from him to the therapist.

Cognitive reframing or providing information can be useful in moderating affect.

Example: In a group struggling with feelings of safety, in part due to change of therapists, the members were expressing their concerns about feeling safe by discussing elements of child care and whether strict discipline would be proper. A schizophrenic member said that he wished his parents had been firmer with him. This comment led to a heated discussion of the cause of mental illness, with patients taking differing stances regarding the weight of biology, upbringing, or parental pathology in the development of their illness. The therapist said that clinicians took all three perspectives into consideration when working with patients. The tension in the room rapidly diminished. The calming effect most likely resulted from the therapist providing information of how he worked, which included containing all three patient perspectives.

Patients' affective engagement in the treatment process is partially determined by the intensity of the resistance to or activation of transferences. Horwitz (1994) observed that groups can both promote and dilute transferences. The therapist's technical approach of neutrality, low structuring, and interpretation (including group-as-a-whole interventions) will intensify transference and stimulation of affect. For patients with severe self and ego deficits, characteristic of the chronically ill, activity, focusing, linking, and remaining in the here and now or future, serve to dilute the intensity of affects and maintain the group as a working entity.

Handling Metaphors

Much communication takes place via metaphors. Patients respond to a stimulus that evokes affect (either consciously or unconsciously), and they comment upon their feelings through metaphors. The most difficult feelings for patients to manage are those stimulated in the transferences and here-and-now interactions within the group. The therapist's tasks are to "hear" and understand the communication and decide in what manner to intervene.

Patients express their feelings about the group in relationship to authority (vertical transferences) and to peers (horizontal transferences). Thus vignettes can be examined in regard to feelings about those in positions of power and responsibility, for example, teachers or bosses as representatives of parents or therapists, or they can be expressed as experiences with schoolmates or coworkers as representatives of siblings and group members. Communications about boundaries may be expressed in terms of dangers in the environment, in public housing, in schools, or in descriptions of recent accidents with injuries. References to peepholes in doors convey need for caution in letting people into one's home (and emotional life). Discussion of physical ailments also communicates members' disabilities or impairments. Often metaphors contain multiple elements, particularly when there is a disturbance within the group that stimulates a wish for the therapist to address problems of safety, bonding, and affect containment.

One of the more frequent metaphors is that of the bus, its occupants, and driver. Like many travel metaphors, the bus represents the therapeutic journey. Unruly students or a passenger out of control contains messages about the state of members' perceptions of the group atmosphere. Descriptions of the driver's behavior in relation to the passengers are frequently a container of unexpressed wishes or hopes that members have in relation to the therapist. A driver was discourteous to passengers, did not stop at a corner, was late, or should have called the police to evict disruptive students. Warm and affectionate feelings about the group may be expressed as friendships with other riders or the driver. One patient developed an adolescent crush on a woman driver as a displacement from his feelings directed to the therapist.

Reality events that are disturbing, such as a therapist's absence, a missed session because of a holiday, or the presence of a new member can be initially addressed in displacement and then more directly explored in relation to the in-group feelings. Patients seem capable of containing emotions stirred by these events and can begin to examine their feelings in a limited way. It is important to appreciate that some of the patients' responses may be compliance with their perceptions of the therapist's messages rather than their more genuine examination of the experience.

Conflicts among members or with the therapist are more difficult to address in the group, but as a group works together over a period of time, the more direct feelings can be examined. Patients should be provided the opportunity to expand their capacity to manage the feelings conveyed through metaphors, but the therapist must also respect their responses, which may signal patients' sense of danger.

Metaphorical communications can be successfully managed in the displacement, and the therapist's understanding of patients' emotional positions can be conveyed through this medium (Katz, 1983). The therapist's task is to understand the metaphor in the transference and then find a way to work within the displacement, listening carefully to members as they "metabolize" the intervention. Specific guidelines to help determine which metaphors might be productively translated into the here and now of the group are unavailable. In insight therapy, interpreting transferences is thought to be essential for change, but many patients make significant gains without specifically exploring their in-group emotional responses. Listening to responses to interventions within the metaphor will inform the clinician. If patients expand on ideas and/or problem solve, it may be unnecessary or counterproductive to translate the metaphor into the group. However, in situations of group boundary disruptions, particularly by the therapist, patients may benefit from the clinician's willingness to examine their responses to the event.

Promoting Problem Solving

One of the therapist's tasks is to assist members in managing their problems of living. Indeed, one of the special attributes of group treatment arises from members' knowledge and everyday experiences of surviving under conditions of bureaucratic regulation and poverty. Many of them are familiar with methods of negotiating with systems that control housing, food stamps, access to medical care and transportation (not all patients have case managers who assist in solving these problems). Even in early stages of group formation, members will give advice to one another, for example, how to obtain food at the free store, or where they might acquire furniture. Simple but valuable suggestions regarding which cab companies help carry groceries up to second and third-floor apartments serve multiple functions in the group, which include bonding members and enhancing feelings that membership can be useful. One member was very appreciative of another's suggestion that she have her bank, where her social security disability checks were deposited, pay her routine bills, because she had been unable to reliably make payments and intermittently her electricity or her cable TV service had been cut off.

Following identification of themes, the clinician might inquire how individuals have managed a situation. Frequent themes that readily lend themselves to this approach are those of disappointments within the family: children forget birthdays; they make promises to visit and then change plans; siblings who have been more successful show off their success; or family gatherings take place and patients are forgotten. Certainly, many themes reflect the "group as family," but the therapist may chose to address the theme in a problem-solving mode by asking how members handle the various situations. The ensuing process often pays rich therapeutic dividends as members provide different responses. The emergence of differences and the group and therapist's capacity to contain those differences, thereby enhancing members' capacity to hear others' opinions, may be a valuable aspect of a problem-solving focus.

As patients explore ways to address problems, they become aware of the satisfaction and increase in self-esteem and self-efficacy that accompany successfully helping others.

> *Example*: The patients in this group were all diagnosed with schizophrenia or schizoaffective disorder, with the exception of Mr. P, a very passive man enmeshed in a symbiotic relationship with his mother. In the context of women exploring unsatisfying relationships, Ms. N described her boyfriend's visual difficulty that limited him to seeing only parts of written documents. However, he had found ways of continuing to work as an accountant. The therapist commented that he had shown considerable persistence in overcoming his impairment and suggested that each of them were also working to overcome problems resulting from their illness.
>
> The subsequent silence was broken by Ms. N commenting how good the cookies were that Ms. M had brought to the session. Mr. P told of giving instruction about bus schedules to strangers, but worrying that he did not do it correctly and scared that he would be attacked by the individuals to whom he was giving directions. The therapist wondered if Mr. P was describing why he was cautious and if he was also cautious in offering ideas in the group. Mr. P answered affirmatively. Mr. Q remarked that it was good to hear Mr. P taking risks, and then he added that he also was cautious.
>
> Mr. Q then asked Ms. N what she thought, and she said she wasn't listening; she was thinking about the cookies. This was followed by a brief discussion between Ms. N and Ms. M about their pleasure in cooking.
>
> Mr. Q then told a story, saying that at the hospital where he volunteered he had run some errands for a doctor who did not have the courtesy even to thank him. Mr. Q continued saying that he learned a lesson that he should be more sensitive to others' feelings. When the therapist commented that Mr. Q had felt hurt, Mr. Q said that it was no big deal. During the remainder of the session, patients examined how they handled feelings when they were not treated with respect.

This example illustrates the nature of members' capacity to examine their successes. The therapist's initial translation of the metaphor to patients overcoming impairments was followed by a seemingly unconnected association, but actually addressed a sector of Ms. M's competence. Mr. P more directly addressed his anxieties, and Mr. Q linked with him in describing his caution. It then appeared that Mr. Q attempted to "recruit" others in joining a subgroup, and when that was unsuccessful (the two women paired around cooking) Mr. Q communicated his displeasure with doctors. In subsequent sessions, Mr. Q was directly able to express his sense of injury with the therapist's use of the word "impairment," which he felt did not recognize the changes he had made in the group. The theme of overcoming disability had partially been derailed as Mr. Q responded to his injury, and yet, over several sessions, he was able to directly express himself, which was an achievement.

The example illustrates how problem solving is not limited to external situations. Members overcome fears and demonstrate, in the here and now changes in their capacities to manage affects. Information emerges as members provide or accept ideas. Do individuals insist that their suggestion be followed? Are useful ideas offered in a manner that provides "space" for the recipient? How are suggestions managed? Are they almost automatically accepted or rejected? Are they thoughtfully considered? In promoting problem solving, psychological work factors (see Chapter 7) of interpersonal input and output and self-under-standing are activated.

What is emphasized in promoting problem solving is not merely a search for concrete solutions. Rather, the treatment process following a focus on problem solving enables therapists to understand patients' inner emotional capacities within a spectrum of group therapeutic factors.

Promoting Self-Understanding (Insight)

Self-understanding is essentially a cognitive process. Insight helps individuals integrate many experiences and place them in a framework that becomes a component of their self-image. This contributes, but is not the sole element, in effecting enduring change. Insight can be broadly conceptualized as learning about oneself across several dimensions, including the sources and impact of affective and behavioral responses. Yalom (1985) observes, "Insight occurs when one discovers something important about oneself—about one's behavior, one's motivational system, or one's unconscious" (p. 46).

In groups significant occasions for learning occur in the immediacy of the here-and-now interactions, in which members can discover stimuli for their responses or their impact on others. The group arena expands patients' opportunities to learn about behaviors and responses in relation to the multiplicity of interactions. In contrast to dyadic treatment in which patients interact solely with the therapist, who most frequently represents an authority or parent, members' engagement is with authority and peers, which broadens potential learning experiences.

Patients' capacities for gaining self-understanding may be limited by their prior experiences or by the degree of their pathology. A person's ability to introspect, to look inside and not focus on external causes as the source of frustration or discomfort may be limited, but change is possible.

Acquisition of new self-understanding often is accompanied by considerable psychic stress. Fears of destructiveness, loss of control, or intense guilt or shame are prominent. At a more archaic level, individuals may suddenly become aware of feelings that their psychic structure (their self) may disintegrate or disappear. It is understandable why anyone would develop a protective screen from such experiences.

In the context of chronically ill patients' vulnerabilities, the therapist has a major task of shaping the group and creating an environment of support and safety in which patients can commence a "risky" encounter with their inner worlds. Seemingly superficial insights may be strongly defended against because of the stress associated with self-reflection.

Many times the initial element in self-learning is a confrontation, offered either by the therapist or a fellow member. The content of the confrontation may be an observation regarding behavior (including physical or emotional components), either as a single element or as a recurrent pattern. The confrontation might simply be a statement of the confrontor's response to the confronted person. The optimal goal of a confrontation is to gently draw the confronted individual's attention to an element in his or her presentation. Confrontations differ from confrontive behavior that is assaultive. Often the confronted person experiences what he or she is told as an assault, which it may be. The therapist then has an additional task of exploring the experience of the confrontor, who may not be aware of any aggressiveness in the statement. Nevertheless, confrontations and confrontative behaviors are part of the fabric of group therapy. Therapists need to keep in mind that even the most benignly intended confrontation may be experienced as intrusive and evoke a self-protective response. Understanding recipients' inner experience, rather than criticizing them for being "too sensitive," will promote the therapeutic relationship and potentially move therapy forward.

Insight can accrue from observing others' behaviors. Patients might remark about seeing aspects of themselves in others' interactions. This mirroring phenomenon is a particular advantage of group treatment. Mirroring can take place with or without verbal input from others. The likelihood of such self-reflection occurring is increased in an accepting and cohesive group.

Insights may not be immediate, but they may suddenly emerge at a time not directly related to a confrontation or an interpretation.

Example: A woman diagnosed with borderline personality with many dependent features frequently would become angry and attack others. The therapists, after observing the process on a number of occasions, began to interpret her anger as a manifestation of her envy of another's being the center of attention.

Several months later this patient interrupted herself in the midst of criticizing a woman and said that she was jealous, just as the therapists had said to her a number of times. On this occasion, the therapists had not made the connection in their own thinking.

In this situation, the insight represents the patient's significant progress in examining her own behavior.

In groups of chronically ill members, most insights are gained in the here and now of the meeting or in relation to current life situations. Clinicians seldom make references to patients' developmental past (family of origin), but some patients will spontaneously bring up childhood experiences in their efforts to further expand and consolidate self-understanding.

It is most useful to offer insight from the perspective of the patient—an empathic understanding of what might contribute to an individual's behavior. To help patients consider that they were withdrawing *because* someone else was the center of attention, or *because* they had hoped for a response that was not forthcoming and felt injured assists in the cognitive processing of an emotional or behavioral response. Not all insight has to be gained from an immediate transaction. The clinician can link prior similar experiences with more here-and-now transactions to help patients gain perspective about both current and prior responses. Some opportunities for gaining self-understanding are achieved when there is some distance, and the emotional temperature is not near the boiling point. Then the therapist can provide an insight that could be more coolly examined and integrated by the patient or the group.

Interventions leading to insight can be offered to the entire group. These may not specifically address each person's response, but may address a particular groupwide response. For example, all members might respond to a vacation, entry of a new member, departure of another, or even a community event. An invitation to explore such happenings may lead most, if not all, present to examine their responses. As with all interpretations or questions inviting patients to consider aspects of their behavior, clinicians should be aware of how their comments are phrased in order to encourage members to offer alternatives or to disagree.

Patients protect themselves in a variety of ways against gaining effective insight that might produce change. A common defensive maneuver is for a patient who has just become aware of a behavioral pattern (via confrontation or interpretation) to inquire, "Why do I do that?" Another response is to comment, "I will change my behavior." A third neutralizing response is to immediately make a connection to a member of the family of origin: "It was because you remind me of my father." The immediacy of such responses (there is no "space" for contemplation) suggests that the patient is fending off "pain" associated with gaining new understanding. Clinicians should begin to explore, usually within themselves first, the basis for the resistance.

The ultimate goal of insight is to effect change in feelings and/or behavior. It is not the only pathway to change, but also acquisition of self-understanding buttresses change that takes place as a consequence of other therapeutic factors. Keeping in mind the differing levels of insight may provide clinicians opportunities to act like a therapist, satisfy their curiosity, and elicit something desirable.

THERAPISTS' STYLE

The seven tasks enumerated for the clinician's attention serve only as a rough map helping to integrate the plethora of information that flows in the members' interaction with their environment, the group, its members, and therapist(s). This framework does not directly address elements of the therapist role that examine style (Rutan & Stone, 1993). Style elements include polarized pairs of activity–nonactivity, transparency–opaqueness, and gratification–frustration. Style is in part implicit in the tasks because the therapist must keep in mind the maintenance of a treatment relationship that helps contain patients' anxieties and allows them to proceed at a pace they can manage in their search for improved internal and external functioning.

Patients are influenced by therapist behavior. They attend to how he or she interacts with them, both verbally and nonverbally. Indeed, often patients perceive the nonverbal channel (including paralinguistic elements) as superordinate, believing that it carries more information about their relationship with the clinician than do words alone. An inactive clinician may convey a willingness to attentively listen to patients, but the same inactivity may be interpreted as disinterest, thereby undermining the relationship. Similarly, therapists are often quite transparent. They emit a variety of nonverbal behaviors that indicate interest or feelings (how they sit in their chair, the degree of eye contact, the encouraging nods, and of course, their facial expressions). Patients will question directly or comment indirectly through metaphors about their therapist's behaviors.

Each clinician will develop a style that is personally comfortable and serves to advance treatment. How opaque or how gratifying each person will be evolves from the person's personality and the patient's needs. Self-awareness and self-scrutiny combined with attention to the treatment process will inform therapists of the impact of their style upon the treatment. Rigid adherence to a particular way of doing things may not serve the therapy.

SUMMARY

In this chapter, characteristics and motivations of therapists have been explored as they are applicable to conducting groups for chronically mentally ill individuals. By gaining awareness of some of their motivations, therapists are in a better position to manage their emotions that inevitably are stimulated in filling the leadership role.

The tasks are enumerated as guidelines and attention to one task impacts upon the others. The therapist's focus at any moment may shift, but recognition that the group acts like an open system in which an intervention at a particular level influences all others, sometimes in quite unpredictable fashion, should provide the clinician with a modicum of intellectual and emotional stimulation. Attention to the treatment process counteracts boredom and disinterest that may overtake even the most highly motivated clinician.

TEN

THE BEGINNING SESSIONS

The meetings themselves represent a social situation, and difficulties of social adaptation which may easily be lost sight of in individual interviews are shown up in sharp relief, particularly when the individual's own particular social difficulties are re-enacted.

—JONES (1948/1972, p. 93)

ollowing completion of the preparatory work, the clinician approaches the first group meeting with relief that the main event is about to begin. Nevertheless, accompanying the excitement is a sense of foreboding. Therapists wonder if anyone will actually attend and if all of the preparatory efforts have gone for naught. One antidote to these anxieties is to send reminders or personally contact all members shortly before the scheduled first meeting. This is particularly useful if the process of forming the group has been prolonged.

Therapists can reflect on their anxieties and consider the emotional position of the prospective members. Optimally, as part of their leadership preparation, therapists will have participated in an unstructured experiential group in which they learned about anxieties and tasks of entering a group. Those experiences should be recalled as they try to empathize with members' anticipatory anxiety.

STRUCTURE

Structure serves to alleviate patients' initial fears, and therapists do well to find ways of containing their own and their patients' anxieties through supplying structure and stimulating participation.

The meeting room should be prepared in advance and seats set up for all who are expected to attend. At the appointed time, patients should be invited into the room (from the waiting area) and the door closed. Receptionists can be provided a membership roster and direct latecomers to proceed to the group room. By beginning promptly, clinicians signal their efforts to create reliable time and space boundaries.

Structuring has two components: (1) restating the agreement and (2) introducing members. The therapist may commence the session with a review of the group agreement, briefly recapping the purposes of the group, reminding members that they have previously established their treatment goals, and restating ground rules of behavior that will create a therapeutic enterprise. Therapists should also include remarks about their own contributions to the treatment. The very process of restating what has been addressed in preparatory sessions indicates that the therapist will participate in the meetings.

The second structuring component is introduction of members. Patients should be asked to introduce themselves, and they can be told that first names will suffice. They are not asked to reveal why they have come to group or to state their goals. Such a request stirs anxiety and may be counterproductive. However, to give one's name means that each person has spoken and the barrier of silence is broken. Following the go-around of names, the therapist can indicate that patients may proceed in any fashion they wish. Such a comment moves the process from one in which the clinician has created a group boundary and defined the work of the group to one in which members are to assume responsibility for what happens.

THE BEGINNING PROCESS

Patients react to the change with varying degrees of anxiety, distrust, and at times markedly regressive behavior. The clinician needs to be alert to the potential for disruptive behaviors or anxiety and yet allow the members sufficient opportunity to interact. The task is to address issues of safety and peer interaction.

Silence of relatively brief actual duration may be experienced as painfully prolonged. In most instances, it is unnecessary for the leader to intervene, and after a short pause, members will begin to talk and begin the process of determining what can be safely exposed in a situation fraught with unknowns. However, if the silence is prolonged, by attempting to engage the members, the clinician demonstrates a willingness to work to promote treatment and help contain affects. Interventions should serve to decrease reverie and maintain interactions in the here and now of the meeting.

Some groups will begin the discussion by attempting to clarify group structures. Members may ask for clarifications of the agreement. They may inquire as to how they should inform the doctor if there is a conflict with the group time and another doctor's appointment, or how they should notify the therapist if they have to miss a meeting because of illness. Others may ask the therapist to provide an agenda. Questions are relatively impersonal, exploring group boundaries and group structures. The therapist demonstrates a willingness to interact by answering such questions: for example, "I don't set up an agenda because I want members to talk about the things that are important to them"; or "Please call the secretary or myself if you cannot be present at a meeting." Therapists' fears that answering questions will inhibit interactions and that patients will flee from self-disclosure by filling the entire session with questions are unfounded. The therapist may also use this initial process to begin to link patients. Comments noting that several members appear to be trying to learn how the group will work serve a linking function.

In most instances, patients will begin cautious self-revelation. This may involve telling where they live or how they were referred to the group. These relatively superficial comments serve to diminish isolation and are often a search for commonalities. Patients may initiate their membership by discussing their illnesses and medications. The topic might be elaborated in a variety of ways that reflect the anxiety of entering the group: Medications cause problematic side effects; doctors have not listened when they were told about problems with medications (which might include direct statements about being given incorrect medications); medications have been particularly helpful; in the hospital, nurses have not been available; they have been frightened by other patients' craziness, violence, or loss of control. Experiences of ostracism or bizarre responses by others to their illness are recounted. These communications convey an underlying sense of demoralization and hopelessness by citing failures of caregivers or peers to be available to understand and respond to them. They also serve to develop a common ground among the patients.

Discussions of family transactions serve as metaphors for the anticipated tasks and problems in joining the group. Members' descriptions of how their families have cared for others include references to being overburdened (fears in the here and now that the therapists will be unable or unwilling to care for them) or to being incompetent. Stories of children's misbehavior and parental rejecting responses are related from personal or hearsay experience, or gleaned from the current news media. Embedded in these vignettes are patients' fears and feelings of uncertainty or helplessness that may be further highlighted as they offer one another suggestions that are rejected as ineffective. Clinicians are not immune to these affects, and they may find themselves responding to the covert pressures to magically find solutions.

At times, patients will speak directly of their fears in anticipation of joining the group. This directness can be addressed by asking for elaboration or by inquiring if those present have similar concerns. Others may begin by indicating that they are looking forward to getting advice from members in managing problems. Rarely is the individual questioned for more details, but the problem is accepted at face value. Responses are provided in concrete terms. Sometimes, respondents merely tell of an analogous episode from their own experiences, an example of parallel talk. Careful attention to these initial discussions will show that the patients are primarily focused on the therapist's response, rather than the impact of their comments on one another, which is characteristic of opening phase behavior.

Therapists should be prepared to listen for metaphorical communication. Sudden switches in topic are not merely distractions, efforts to contain anxiety, or manifestations of self-absorption, but may represent a communication about the developing therapeutic process.

> *Example*: Following the review of the agreement and members introducing themselves in a go-around in the first meeting of a coled group, two members spoke directly of feeling anxious because they were meeting strangers. This led to several tales of frightening experiences, including hearing a minister describe how he had to exorcise demons from a mentally ill person. That vignette was followed by a change of tone in the session from anxiety to sadness, and members discussing how they felt different and alone. This theme was summarized by one of the therapists, who added that it was certainly expectable for people entering a group to feel some uncertainty about how they were going to join a group of strangers.
>
> A white woman offered some hope when she related that although she had been rejected by her family, she had been adopted by a black woman who had cared for her. Another woman said that a lot of people did not understand mental illness, and she was glad there were efforts to educate the public and help reduce some of the stigma and isolation. A man concluded the meeting by describing his determination to keep going despite his anxiety, and working had proven to be supportive.

The cotherapists had limited their interventions to indicating their understanding of the manifest content of the members' associations, inquiring if others had something to add to what had been said, and summarizing themes. The process suggested that direct expression of anxiety in meeting strangers evoked fears that their inner demons would be exposed. The shift in affect suggested that they had isolated themselves to protect against exposing their demons, but that solution had as concomitant a sense of aloneness. The therapist's intervention, making their discussion understandable and expectable, shifted the mood, and hope emerged.

As the first session draws to a close, the therapist might again make contact with members who have remained silent and inquire if they wish to add anything to the discussion. A patient's ability to participate in early group sessions has been predictive of his or her remaining in the group. Failure of patients to participate may be experienced as a confirmation of their personal deficits or their inability to interact with others, and result in dropping out (MacKenzie, 1994). It is therefore necessary to decide whether to summarize the proceedings. It may be useful to recap the themes and the anxieties that have been expressed and indicate the typical nature (if accurate) of the issues that have been addressed. This provides members with a sense that the therapist has understood what has happened, and it also provides closure. However, summarizing the sessions should not become a routine procedure, because it may reinforce passivity by inviting patients to wait for "the word" at the end of a session. Therapists also should be cautious about overstating the positive nature of the meeting. Patients have had many experiences of relationships starting positively only to be disappointed. The clinician does well not to promise what cannot be delivered. Therapists may close by indicating that they are looking forward to seeing the members at the next session.

Several goals should be achieved by the close of the first session. The therapist must attempt to prevent members from exposing themselves in a fashion that will result in their feeling isolated, frightened, or disillusioned to the extent that they will not return. They should depart with a sense that they can achieve something from belonging to the group. This may be accomplished by helping members link either with subgroups or the whole membership. If possible, no person should be left as a singleton. The summary, with a mention of each member's participation, may accomplish this goal. In addition, the therapist, in his or her interactions by listening and responding, begins to serve as a model for identification (Kennard, 1993).

EARLY SESSIONS

Patients' central concerns of trust, safety, and intimacy emerge during the early meetings. Seldom are these issues discussed directly, but they are communicated through metaphors or actions. Therapists are faced with the difficult task of listening to what members say and how they interact and tell their stories, and finding ways of intervening that will appreciate the patients' vulnerabilities. This must be accomplished while maintaining respect for patients' strengths and capacities to alter earlier experiences of distrust, danger, and callousness.

Trust is not a given. It must be earned. Members have had many experiences of betrayal that may be deeply ingrained, and only gradually will they put their feet in the water. They worry that they will be pulled into a maelstrom in which others act unreliably. Patients try to determine if the therapist will be trustworthy. They may tell stories of unreliable parents, failures of transportation services, public officials, or police being rude or hostile as communications about what they may expect to happen or what has already transpired in relation to those in authority as stand-ins for the therapist(s). Distrust of peers may be conveyed in stories of failures of friends or neighbors. This distrust may be enacted when members ask about last names or phone numbers and there is no response. Careful observation will reveal that some individuals back away from revealing more personal information. Behaviors before and after the meeting also provide data as to members' evolving trust. Who sits together in the waiting area? What transpires there? Who comes late? What subgrouping takes place following the meeting? Answers to these questions require a certain amount of inference, but therapists should be alert to behaviors as they build a mental image of each person's abilities to interact in a trusting fashion.

Discussion of religion may reflect important aspects of trust. Can one put trust in God? Is the church the only place where one can have faith? Members may express considerable differences in their discussion of religion. For some, church is a place where they feel accepted; and for others, it represents a place of considerable cynicism. Often religious topics are introduced into the treatment process when there has been a disappointment in the group. Patients can easily become engaged in discussion of a pastor, women's activities, or of God as a way of communicating that another setting is more trustworthy (or safe) than that of the group.

> *Example*: A meeting began with a member telling of attending a funeral for a relative who had committed suicide. Another member responded by recalling having gone to a funeral of a young man studying for the ministry who also had committed suicide. This led to a discussion of religion and various aspects of the Bible and church life that members enjoyed. The therapist suggested that suicides were often unknowable and religion might help us understand. Several patients agreed, and one man added that he felt that the discussion of religion had been really good, because in many places similar talk led to major disagreements or were not allowed.

The patients' experience of comradery in discussing their relationships with religion as a response to the stress of hearing about suicide strengthened the group bonds. Although not addressed directly in this segment, the discussion created an opportunity to examine members' hidden aspects of themselves that are difficult to share.

Safety issues are of major importance not only in the beginning phases but also throughout the life of the group. Safety may be thought of from the position of the consequences of group interaction. In the broadest sense, what are the risks and how might one be injured, either through the actions of others or through one's loss of control? Certainly physical safety is of fundamental importance. Threats to act on feelings need to be contained, and firm limits set. Patients need to be told clearly that they cannot inflict physical harm on others. In the interpersonal setting of a group, it is easy to lose sight of a disturbed member's struggle to contain his or her feelings and actions. The therapist's intervention not only protects the group, but also functions to reassure the individual on the verge of losing control that the therapist will work to keep things safe. For instance, an unstable bipolar patient may respond to the stimulation of the group with progressive excitement and agitation. Firm efforts to deal with this situation are necessary to protect the patient's present and future relationship with others. At times, it may be necessary to ask a person to leave the room, not as a punishment, but as an opportunity for him or her to regain composure.

Emotional safety is fundamental to group progress. Patients are not given license to express their feelings through attacks on others. Inevitably, differences emerge that will touch vulnerable sectors of each others' personalities. The result may be critical or angry outbursts, or the response may be metaphors in which individuals are mugged, robbed, or their homes broken into. These interactions provide an opportunity for therapists to clarify acceptable ways of self-expression. At the same time, the therapist can try to understand the precipitant for the aggressive person's behavior.

Withdrawal is a more frequent response to disagreement, generally having arisen from members' developmental (family) experiences of having the expression of feelings frowned upon, if not outrightly criticized. Yet from the perspective of emotional safety, a patient who puts forth a feeling or an idea and is responded to with silence receives the message that it is unsafe to express such emotions. The injury potentially sets in motion a downward spiral of mutual withdrawal in the service of safety.

The therapist may find it necessary to interact with the individual who has not received a response. Here, the issue of timing becomes important, because premature interventions by the clinician may deprive others, who did not initially react, of the opportunity to comment. Patients do not gain quite the same boost in self-esteem when they follow the leader, in contrast to situations in which they speak first.

Many patients quite consciously test the group situation by only revealing part of a story and dangling clues that there is more. In early stages of group development, members' own anxieties may interfere with their responding, and they also may be testing to see if the therapist will protect them. Clinical judgment is necessary to assess members' therapeutic alliance, which would enable them to explore their own withdrawal response. Frequently, those interventions are best deferred until a more solid treatment relationship has been established.

Closely linked with issues of trust and safety are those of intimacy. Patients seldom directly express their wishes for a close, enduring, warm relationship. Rather, themes of irresponsibility, abandonment, and loss convey the feared consequences of forming an intimate friendship. A direct communication of members' capacities to engage and to form close attachments is expressed in their attendance. The flexibly bound model legitimizes patients' struggles to belong to a group and yet maintain a distance that is manageable. The option of altering one's agreement allows the patient to be the accepted locus of control.

> *Example*: In the ninth group meeting, the therapist observed that all those present had contracted to attend weekly. Ms. E corrected him, saying she would miss occasionally because she had to care for her elderly mother. Ms. M told how she felt good when she cooked meals for an ill friend. Ms. A said she was no longer interested in going to church regularly, even though she liked the people. Ms. M expressed ambiguous feelings, describing how much everyone hugged and kissed, but wondering how genuine they were and citing that no one had called her when she had been ill for a month. Ms. A told how she hated cooking, but feared her husband's wrath if she expressed her resentment. Mr. D told how he would take stands against his family members, but they would describe him as ungrateful.

The therapist's opening remark appeared to stimulate considerable anxiety about the meaning of attending each session. The associations revealed several patients' wishes to maintain control by being in the role of caregiver. These were followed by an expression of distrust of others' motives (as experienced in the church), and finally more direct fears of the consequences of self-assertion.

The example also expresses concerns about interpersonal and group boundaries. Intimacy is frightening, because one cannot be certain about the motivations of others. However, deeper terrors are hinted at by reminders that members would not regularly attend the group or their church. The sequence suggests that members do not feel that they can reliably "open and close" their personal boundaries, and they respond to what might be experienced as a demand for intimacy (the observation that they all had agreed to attend weekly) by a discussion of stepping outside the group boundary. Even though it appeared that a core subgroup had formed, the tentative nature of this achievement was expressed in the associations and the absence of two of the five participants in the succeeding session.

GROUP BOUNDARIES

Not all early sessions go smoothly. Therapists are faced with a number of vexing behaviors that may become normative if they do not receive attention. The behaviors might be addressed within a conceptual framework of internal and external group boundaries.

The group agreement specifies flexibility in the frequency with which patients may attend meetings, but the agreement is explicit about attending on time and remaining throughout the entire session. Obviously, this portion of the agreement is frequently ignored. Patients do not invariably explain the reason for their lateness, and if they do, the explanations may be plausible but superficial. Lateness may represent patients' tests to determine if others are genuinely interested in them, or it may be a response to actual or anticipated injury within the group. If inadequate transportation is stated as the reason in some circumstances, alternatives might be suggested (Spotnitz, 1957).

> *Example*: Natalie often missed or came late to sessions. She explained that the trip to the clinic required a lengthy bus trip that entailed a transfer. However, it was evident that she arose in sufficient time, because she helped her child get ready for school. Rather than drop from group treatment, Natalie was transferred to another group, meeting at a more convenient hour. In this setting, Natalie attended in a timely fashion. However, it became evident that the group composition had been a more important influence on her attendance than the transportation. The second group included only two men who attended irregularly, whereas, in the first group, men were in the majority. In the second group, Natalie felt freer to explore her anger with and fears of men.

The clinician had been unaware of the intensity of Natalie's fears, which were further hidden by her initial verbal reticence. It was only after several months in the new group that she was able to discuss these feelings.

Clinical management of patients' late arrival is not simple. The therapist should remain alert to the group response, and if members do not acknowledge the person's presence, then the therapist should do so. For someone coming late to their first meeting, brief introductions will serve to acknowledge their entry; a restatement of the agreement can wait until the end of the session.

An additional consideration is the value of providing a brief summary of the session or of the most recent topic to aid the latecomer to integrate into the session. The temptation to summarize a meeting may represent a countertransference wish to include the member or it may represent a clinically valid response. Each situation requires careful assessment by the clinician before he or she decides to intervene. Patients will respond to inconsistencies in how this is managed, which can be addressed in the ongoing process.

When greater group engagement has been achieved, reasons for, and meaning of, the lateness may be productively explored, but forbearance is indicated in the opening meeting(s).

The mirror image of patients arriving late are those members who leave sessions prematurely. Sometimes patients bolt from the room. At other times, they ask for permission to leave, without providing an explanation, such as "I need to go to the bathroom." If the group is co-led and the patient seems particularly distraught, one of the clinicians might decide to follow the person and attempt to determine the nature of his or her emotional state. A few minutes of contact may clarify the basis for the departure. Efforts to persuade the person to return to the meeting should be sensitive to the individual's vulnerability and capacity to manage his or her affects. In initial stages of singly led groups, unless there is strong evidence for the departing member being severely out of control, the therapist should not leave the group to attend to an individual.

If patients ask permission to leave, a gentle inquiry asking if they can remain may be met with "I will be back in a few minutes." The therapist has expressed interest through such inquiry, and in the process reinforced several norms—those of patient autonomy and the agreement to remain in the meeting for the duration of each session.

Even in the initial session, the remaining members will indirectly respond to these departures. The underlying dynamics of safety, trust, and engagement are stimulated, and they usually are addressed in metaphor. The clinician should silently explore the dynamics precipitating the departure and store that information for future reference. Alternatively, the departure may be addressed in the here and now either directly or using members' metaphors. It is useful to consider the departing member as carrier of a group role (a wish to remove oneself from a stressful situation) that is expressed in a vulnerable individual.

Another boundary crossing takes place when a patient brings a child to the group. Sometimes this is an expression of commitment to the group, but it may also represent a patient's narcissism ("Please admire this offspring") or anxieties about engagement (the child might serve as a distraction). Older children might safely wait in a supervised place (with a receptionist serving as supervisor); infants and young children may be allowed to remain. If possible, there should be sufficient flexibility to enable the patient to remain for the session. Considerable tact is necessary to find a way to explore alternatives the patient might have had to bringing the child. Merely raising the question, however, has the potential for injuring the patient, who may respond by withdrawing or absenting him- or herself from succeeding sessions. However, to ignore addressing the options suggests that the therapist will avoid certain topics, which is not a desirable model for identification. In the end, inquiring about options may be sufficient to carry the message that it would be preferable not to have children present.

The boundaries among members (internal boundaries) and those between the group and external environment both come into focus when a patient is on the verge of losing control. Individuals in the midst of a psychotic decompensation or under the influence of drugs or alcohol may quickly convey their emotional state in the group. Often a reverberating and escalating process takes place in the interactions, overstimulating everyone. The therapist must weigh individual and group needs. On balance, protecting the group and promoting a sense of safety should take precedence. Thus, if a patient is unable to be contained in the meeting, then he or she should be asked to leave. At times, an explanation that the group seems to be very stimulating suffices for a person to depart the meeting. The person also could be asked to wait so that the therapist can meet with him or her after the session is finished. Obviously, in the case of a major emergency, the particular patient's needs should take precedence, but this would occur infrequently.

Within the meeting, the boundary of the group circle may be altered by patients who express their anxieties by moving their seats outside the circle. A gentle invitation to join the circle may suffice to let the patient know that the behavior has been noted. Insistence that a person more actively participate, either by moving his or her chair into the circle or by speaking is contraindicated (see example in Chapter 13). The therapist can be assured that a part of each member wishes to flee from the novel experience, and the "deviant" behavior represents both an individual and a group role. In some instances, addressing fears others may have regarding engagement will serve to lower anxiety, and the patient may spontaneously rejoin the circle.

The boundary between members becomes problematic when monopolization takes place. Even recognizing that, in part, a monopolizer relieves others from having to reveal themselves and members may have participated in the process, the therapist must appreciate that it is unlikely that, particularly early in treatment, members will be able to effectively interrupt the process. The therapist then must ask the monopolizer to provide others an opportunity to talk and reinforce that pronouncement if necessary. Even though monopolization may have been a product of group interactions, patients will feel shortchanged if time has not been provided for them to talk.

Some members fail to cross the boundary into the group by not attending sessions. The therapist can review the group roster and attempt to contact individuals who had been expected to attend. A phone contact may be an expression of sufficient interest that an ambivalent patient will risk coming to the next meeting. This may be a useful procedure to continue, keeping in mind that patients may manage their need for emotional space through their behavior. Following a member's attending four sessions and reaching agreement regarding the frequency of attendance, therapists may use attendance charts (see Chapter 11) to monitor compliance. The therapist must decide whether to promptly contact patients after they fail to attend a session or wait and see how a person will manage his or her agreement.

TRANSFERENCE

Patients enter treatment with expectations and distortions from prior interpersonal encounters. These expectations from the past, brought into the present, are the essence of transference. The psychoanalytic setting, with the analyst's position out of the patient's view, is an effort to minimize external stimuli. When that is linked to the analyst's neutrality, the treatment situation is thought to be optimal for patients to reexperience their past distortions or developmental fixations. However, Freud (1905), in his earliest formulations, recognized that transferences occur in everyday life and are not limited to the analytic situation.

Gradually the notion of the therapist as a blank screen onto which patients would project their expectations and fears was replaced by a more interactive model in which therapists' behaviors (verbal and nonverbal) were acknowledged as contributing to patients' perceptions (Greenberg & Mitchell, 1983). Recognition of the interactive nature of treatment shifted focus into the here-and-now transactions. Kohut (1971, 1977, 1984) expanded understanding of transferences in his formulations of the psychology of the self, with its emphasis on a person's lifelong need for another to fulfill self-stabilizing functions (selfobjects). Elucidation of selfobject transferences provided a theoretical buttress to the clinical awareness of the impact of patient–therapist interactions and of narcissistic vulnerabilities.

Group psychotherapy pioneers translated the dyadic situation into the group and focused on patients' transferences to the therapist as the central dynamic force (Slavson, 1957; Wolf, 1968). Members were conceptualized as available to serve as displacements for the therapist or as representatives of siblings (Aronson, 1975).

In addition to individual transferences, members were found to develop internalized images of the group as a whole, which could be equated to early parental images (Bion, 1961; Durkin, 1964; Slater, 1966; Scheidlinger, 1974). These images portrayed the group as harsh and destructive, as a place of refuge and safety, or as a combination of the two. The notion of the group as a whole then added a significant dimension to the conceptualization of patients' experiences and thereby increased the complexity of understanding patients' inner worlds.

Perceptions of the group leader may be quite diverse. Some patients might see the therapist as warm and protective and as a source of salvation from the dangers of the group. Their mothers may have been overprotective. Others may respond to the therapist as cold and withholding, as they had to their own psychotic mothers. Still others may experience the therapist in the opening sessions as disinterested, like their fathers who were never at home. The diversity of responses that arise from members focusing on their experience of salient aspects of the therapist represents everyday transferences (Klein, 1977).

Transferences also are evident when there is uniformity of members' perspectives about the group, the leader, or a particular individual. The lack of differences indicates the presence of powerful feelings that can not be critically assessed. The patients treat the situations as real and have considerable difficulty in maintaining a differentiation in cognitive and experiencing aspects of the ego (Ashback & Schermer, 1987, p. 186).

Many individuals resist exposing their expectations or responses to others, consciously and unconsciously. They maintain their distance because of the personal meaning entailed in exposing earlier developmental needs or conflicts. For instance, a person may fear losing his or her personal integrity and being engulfed by the image of the group, thereby losing a sense of self. Others may feel that expressing childish feelings is shameful and, as a consequence, maintain barriers to engagement. As a generalization, seriously ill individuals have experienced significant interpersonal trauma in the past, and they are particularly cautious about exposing themselves in the present, where their needs and wishes might again be frustrated or ignored. It is such resistance that often plays such a prominent role in members' responses to entering a group.

Groups provide multiple opportunities to explore experiences of engagement and separation. Patients may express their anxieties by not attending, coming late, maintaining emotional distance, or monopolizing attention out of fear that without attention they will suffer abject aloneness.

Management of these relationship distortions is intertwined with the therapist's tasks in the beginning stages of group formation. Patients' responses to the clinician's interventions managing boundaries, bonding, or identifying affect may be considered as transference manifestations. For instance, if a therapist attempts to link one person with another, and the patient "resists," then the response might be understood as the patient's experience of the therapist as controlling, or as fear of intimacy or joining, or as a realistic response to the therapist's inaccurate basis for making the link.

It is not always easy to recognize interpersonal expressions of each member's developmental arrests or conflicts. They may emerge either rapidly or slowly in the therapeutic process. If a particular need or interpersonal response is important in a patient's psychology, it will appear in different forms and at different times, which will provide the clinician with multiple opportunities for its detection and possible resolution.

COUNTERTRANSFERENCE

Therapists experience a broad range of emotions in leading groups. Some feelings are not consciously perceived but influence the clinician's response to a particular patient or to the treatment. Such responses have been labeled "countertransference," and as such have been conceptualized as interfering with treatment (Freud, 1910, 1915). This classical view was found to be limiting, and the notion of countertransference has expanded to include the totality of the clinician's emotional responses in the treatment situation (Kernberg, 1975; Roth, 1990). This expanded definition has served an important function in allowing therapists to consider their emotional responses as information about the therapeutic situation. Responses in the clinician may arise from feelings that are induced by patients in their unconscious efforts to communicate aspects of themselves (Racker, 1968). Proper management by the therapist opens the door to understanding patients in greater depth. This expanded perspective on countertransference has vitiated the more narrow and pejoratively tinged assessment that having feelings was an indicator that one was doing something wrong.

Not all therapeutic errors are due to countertransference. A lack of familiarity with certain situations may lead therapists to err. A neophyte clinician may not know how to address certain enactments or may not be familiar with problems, such as a patient bringing a small child to the group under circumstances in which the alternative was to remain home and miss the meeting. As a clinician gains experience, a wide range of situations are more readily managed without disrupting the treatment.

There are relatively few channels for therapists to recognize their unconscious responses. The group agreement provides a useful framework in which some countertransferences can be brought to light. The clinician who is late to the meeting, allows the session to extend beyond the agreed stopping time, or forgets to announce a forthcoming vacation until the last moment can utilize those slips as a signal to look for unrecognized feelings about specific members or the group. If he or she chooses to keep the door open past the specified starting time, until several members milling in the hall come in, then that action should be explored.

If there are significant changes in group interactions that are not readily explainable (and sometimes such explanations can be facile), then a search for countertransferences contributing to this state should be undertaken. Illustrative of such changes would be when a previously verbally active group becomes relatively silent, the therapist experiences drowsiness, or patients make requests following each session.

One strategy for gaining a perspective on countertransference is to review roles patients have taken in the group. Patients who have become the therapist's favorite or who have become those the therapist would like to have leave the group have evoked feelings in the clinician that may have gone unnoticed. Through gaining awareness of these feelings and analyzing the particular role a patient fills, the therapist may be able to understand an aspect of his or her responses that interfered with therapeutic movement.

Example: A therapist reviewing his group in the aforementioned manner recognized that he wished that a particularly narcissistic woman would not return to the group. With this information, he began to explore in more detail the nature of her group interactions. Although she was bright and articulate, on most occasions her behavior was such that she immediately associated to others comments with a story about abuse she received from her wealthy sister and her fears that if she didn't go along with her sister's requests, she would have no one to depend on. The therapist began to examine his own life experiences and rather promptly found his thoughts centering on his own self-absorbed mother. He was then able to listen more to the patient and attempt to find ways to link the themes in the patient's experiences with her sister to those of others, thereby making some headway into her greater integration into the group.

A valuable window into countertransference responses is the clinician's dreams. Dreams, particularly those immediately preceding or following a session, may contain helpful information that can remove therapeutic blocks.

Example: In supervision, a therapist told of a woman member reporting bizarre and frightening behaviors of tenants in her apartment and her wish to be rid of the offenders. The supervisor wondered if this was a communication about the member's fears of exposing similar ideas or feelings in the group. In response, the female cotherapist reported that following the last session she dreamt that the clinic director had come to her and told her to transfer a man, known to be violent, from the group to individual therapy. The supervisor suggested that the dream was linked to the therapist's concerns over expressions of violence or psychotic material. The cotherapists then recalled how the preceding week a patient had come to group on crutches following a car accident, and group themes had included bizarre expressions of snakes biting and attacking, and stories of strange experiences. The supervisor then helped the therapists consider the metaphorical communications and strategies for translating the associations into ordinary language that would help members discuss their in-group fears. This intervention proved successful.

In this example, the therapist's dream helped to focus more sharply on cotherapists' anxieties of violent and psychotic behavior erupting, which interfered with their ability to listen to metaphors and use the information in a therapeutic manner.

The broader definition of countertransference frees clinicians to utilize feelings in the service of understanding members or the group situation (Rutan & Stone, 1993). Therapists have responses almost from the beginning of group interactions. They may be very pleased with the members' interactions, or they may find themselves frustrated with patients' difficulties in interacting, or with the relatively slow progress of a meeting. They may have a model of therapeutic growth that links free exchange of in-group feelings to their own success as clinicians, and as a consequence feel pressure to move the treatment process along. Boredom and dread of sitting through another session are manifestations of failed therapeutic aspirations. A not uncommon countertransference response is the feeling that members will just have to work this out for themselves, an emotional response that should serve as a signal to the therapist.

Some clinicians find themselves compensating for such feelings by becoming overly active. They may find themselves altering their style and "teaching" patients new ways of interacting. They may institute role playing when that has not been part of their usual armamentarium as a way to increase members' engagement. Such changes may be quite effective, but clinicians must concomitantly try to determine if such style changes represent an action on their own feelings.

Therapists' affective responses may be as recipients of patients' projections of their emotional states. A clinician's fears of being attacked or injured, being devoured by oral needs, or overwhelmed by hopelessness may be induced by a single patient or by the entire group (Klein et al., 1990). Such feelings may be mirrors of the members' inner states. Not uncommonly, a considerable segment of a meeting will be consumed with patients citing frustrating experiences in dealing with government bureaucracies, unresponsive landlords, or lengthy waits in medical clinics. The clinician may experience a range of feelings—from frustration, hopelessness, or anger—that is induced by the patients. It is a method of communicating their emotional states.

On occasion even more dramatic examples of patients communicating their affective states arise.

> *Example*: In preparation for a change of therapists coinciding with a transition in training and coincidental with the therapist introducing herself to the members, a severely ill young man brought his pet alligator to the group. During the meeting, the alligator thrashed around in its box and at one moment poked its head out into the room. The patient assured everyone that it would not get out of its container.
>
> The therapists experienced a multitude of feelings, including dismay, terror, and anger. The patient had effectively communicated aspects of himself—his own inner fears of destructiveness linked to the loss of a well-liked physician, and his uncertainty that the incoming clinician would be unable to contain those elements in himself.

Many persistently and seriously mentally ill individuals have developed effective mechanisms for maintaining their distance, and provocative behaviors are among their more successful strategies. Failure to attend meetings or arriving almost at the end of a session with what may seem the clear intent of being present only to obtain medication are frequently irritating behaviors. Negative symptoms of schizophrenia (apathy, social inactivity, withdrawal) also are magnets for feelings of irritation, and are stimuli for high expressed emotion (Runions & Prudo, 1983). Therapists' boredom, withdrawal, and apathy are likely induced feelings that provide a window into patients' emotional states.

It is important that clinicians not allow themselves to be abused. Excessive phone calls or demands for medication or extra care can be brushed aside as arising from a patient's needs that do not require gratification; or they may be responded to by rejecting the patient. Such transactions should be considered part of a patient's communication about his inner state, but limits need to be established. Similarly, patients cannot abuse one another. Accepting a patient's premise that the group is a place where feelings can be expressed without regard for others sets up sadistic–masochistic encounters that are nonproductive and may lead to group destruction.

> *Example*: One woman with a diagnosis of schizoaffective disorder entered the group with a reputation of annoying her caregivers to the point of distraction. The referring clinician hoped that the group would be able to set limits and help her gain an understanding of her impact on others.
>
> Very quickly the patient took control of the group and offered dogmatic opinions about how to manage all problems. Limit setting was difficult, and the therapist sought outside consultation in trying to contain his anger with the patient. The consultation helped him address some of the fragments of information that were present in the patient's verbalizations, hinting at her underlying terror of being abused in relationships. With this assistance, the therapist was able to more effectively understand the patient while continuing to try to set limits. The effect was that the patient described for the first time her rage at her mother for using her to care for 10 younger siblings, while "Mother sat on her ass eating bon bons and smoking cigarettes."
>
> This historical perspective partially altered the members responses, and the patient felt more accepted. She subsequently modified, to the extent she was able, her response to anticipating that others in the group would take advantage of her, and at times she was spontaneously able to stop herself from talking.

In this example, an experienced clinician reacted to the patient's provocations and found himself having difficulty serving as an effective container and also protecting the group. Consultation helped reverse a process that might have destroyed the group and merely repeated the patient's prior experiences of rejection.

Supervision and/or consultation is often necessary to assist therapists in regaining their balance. Even with the knowledge that their affects are useful in understanding group transactions, therapists may be unable to hear communications leading to the source of difficult behavior. Under sway of intense feelings, clinicians have considerable difficulty with cognitively processing information.

SUMMARY

In this chapter, the beginning treatment processes are addressed. Therapists are alerted to the functions of structure as an initial process of creating a safe environment. Patients enter the group with a variety of conscious and unconscious strategies to determine if group will be safe.

They use prior experiences to make linkages and diminish the sense of aloneness, and they are simultaneously mindful of the input from the therapist, who they hope will protect and guide them. Therapists' goals for the initial sessions are discussed in the context of examining elements of trust, safety, and intimacy. Problems in creating a therapeutic environment are examined in a framework of external and internal group boundaries.

Manifestations of transferences, either to the therapist, members, or the group as a whole are examined. Historical and contemporary formulations of countertransference are reviewed. Clinicians are alerted to ways of detecting countertransference that are not fully conscious, and to the use of their own affects in the therapeutic process.

ELEVEN

THE GROUP CENSUS
Attendance, Newcomers, Dropouts, and Terminations

The theory treats any enterprise or institution, or a part of any enterprise or institution, as an open system. Such a system must exchange materials with its environment in order to survive. The difference between what it imports and what it exports is a measure of the conversion activities of the system.

—RICE (1969, p. 566)

In this chapter, three common issues related to influencing group census will be addressed: (1) monitoring attendance, (2) adding members, (3) dropouts and terminations. Groups using the flexibly boundaried model may be subject to considerable variation in attendance as members contract to attend at varying intervals. In addition, inevitably some patients never become engaged in treatment and drop out rather promptly, whereas others seem to disappear more gradually. Clinicians leading groups drawn from the chronically ill population have a more complex task of monitoring the group census than do those conducting more typical outpatient groups.

ATTENDANCE

Within a reasonable time frame, some groups develop a pattern in which attendance at meetings ranges from six to eight patients, and over a period of time, a considerable degree of stability and member relatedness emerges. The pattern in these groups is a regularly attending core group of three or four members, a subgroup of individuals that attend half the time, and a third subgroup who attend either less frequently or erratically. Other groups seem to have less stable patterns and suffer dropouts, falling attendance, and the addition of new members is necessary to sustain the enterprise.

In many situations, maintaining a flowchart of patient and therapist attendance that is readily available for easy perusal will simplify the clinician's tracking patterns of core and peripheral membership as well as reactions to interruptions (e.g., holidays) and therapist absences (Figure 11.1). With a large membership roster and variable attendance agreements, individuals may miss several meetings, come less frequently than agreed upon, or even drop out before the clinician becomes fully aware of what has taken place. Even in settings in which patients are sent reminders after missing a scheduled session, keeping track of 12–16 members can be problematic.

Clinicians are often startled when they observe attendance patterns revealed in attendance charts. A patient who agrees to come once a month may soon be found to have been present only once every 8–10 weeks. Initially hesitant individuals may show an extended pattern of intermittent attendance and then gradually join a solid core group. The change may coincide with the disappearance of a difficult member. Sometimes therapists realize that a quiet person has been present at almost every meeting and yet verbally contributes very little. Some patients will miss blocks of time because of periods of hospitalization, absence from the community, immobilizing stress in their environment, or a reaction to group interactions that cannot be directly addressed and is managed by withdrawal.

In some circumstances, patients may exhibit their ambivalent resistance by notifying the clinic of their forthcoming absence and simultaneously providing a variety of reasons for missing, such as failures of transportation, need to care for relatives or friends' children, or an appointment for a medical problem. In this manner, patients maintain contact, and the clinician may not be as aware of their absence. Moreover, patients diminish the risk of becoming engaged in feared conflictual interactions. They may spontaneously return or only come back after direct outreach.

In addition to monitoring individual attendance, review of broader trends in group attendance is equally revealing. Over extended time periods, core members may attend less frequently, resulting in a decrease in average attendance. If new members have been added, increasing the group census, the number of members present weekly may remain stable, and the change in status from core to peripheral membership might not

FIGURE 11.1. Group attendance record.

NAME	DIAG-NOSIS*	JANUARY				FEBRUARY				MARCH					APRIL			
		4	11	18	25	1	8	15	22	1	8	15	22	29	5	12	19	26
Ms. A	P				✓						✓							
Ms. B	P		✓						✓			✓					✓	
Ms. C	A	✓									✓							
Mr. D	P	✓	✓	✓	✓	✓			✓	✓		✓		✓	✓	✓		
Ms. E	S	✓		✓								✓			✓			✓
Ms. F	S				✓										✓	✓		
Mr. G	S																	
Ms. H	S	✓	✓	✓	✓	✓	✓		✓	✓	✓	✓	✓	✓	✓	✓	✓	✓
Ms. I	S									✓							✓	✓
Ms. J	A, P		✓	✓		✓	✓			✓	✓		✓	✓	✓	✓		
Ms. K	M	✓	✓	✓	✓	✓				✓	✓	✓	✓	✓	✓	✓	✓	
Mr. L	S					✓												
Ms. M	A, P		✓			✓			✓		✓		✓		✓			✓
Ms. N	A	✓	✓		✓						✓	✓						✓
Ms. O	A		✓				✓			✓					✓			✓
Ms. P	A	✓				✓					✓							
Ms. Q	A				✓				✓				✓				✓	
Ms. R	S				✓	✓				✓	✓	✓	✓		✓	✓		
Mr. S	S	✓		✓	✓	✓					✓	✓	✓			✓		
Mr. T	S	✓		✓							✓							
ATTENDANCE		9	7	8	9	9	3		7	7	7	9	8	5	7	7	6	7

*P, Personality disorder; A, affective disorder; S, schizophrenia/schizoaffective disorder. No group on February 15.

be noticed. Clinicians may ignore a decrease in average attendance from seven to six or five persons, but decreases in which there are frequent sessions with less than four patients are not easily disregarded.

It is not unusual for therapists to minimize or deny changes in attendance. They may hope that members who have disappeared will return, or they may feel burdened by the task of recruiting and preparing newcomers. Clinicians often link their self-esteem to their ability to engage patients in treatment, and a falling census may need to be denied in order to maintain therapists' emotional balance. It is sometimes quite discouraging to feel that a group that was so difficult to get started is on the brink of collapse.

A less common but important countertransferential response is represented by the therapist who has been overwhelmed by the leadership responsibilities and has subtly sabotaged the group with the hope of being relieved of the treatment "burden." This becomes a crisis requiring prompt consultation.

More objective data provided by an attendance flowchart bring the situation more sharply into awareness. We have found it useful to review flowcharts quarterly. Significant events can be added to these charts to further elucidate the treatment process. Notation on the record of a cotherapist's absence or of a disruptive event in the meeting may be ample explanation for a sudden decrease in attendance. Records extending for several years may show patterns in response to changes in therapist. An overview of several years can be very salutary for clinicians who can observe indicators of members' engagement.

NEW MEMBERS

Adding members to an ongoing group stimulates continuing patients' anxieties about meeting strangers. Seldom is the prospect anticipated with a positive tinge that a newcomer will add to the group interaction. Instead, primarily in metaphor, the experience is envisioned as one of deprivation rather than an opportunity to learn new ways of managing stranger anxiety. When the group census is severely diminished, newcomers may be accepted as a way of keeping the group alive, and the "person" of the incoming individual is of secondary importance. These reactions represent both the members' anxieties in meeting strangers and their overt and covert attachments to the status quo.

In the early phase of treatment, it may be useful to inform the group about the desired census and that new members may be attending in the first several weeks. Despite the relative instability of membership, members may develop surprisingly strong feelings not only about absences but also about newcomers.

Example: Angela, diagnosed with schizoaffective disorder, entered the third session of a newly formed group in which additional members had entered at each meeting. Four members were present, and three members who had been present during the preceding sessions were absent. A person who had been announced had changed her mind and did not start in the group. Following the therapist's review of the agreement and introduction of Angela, René agitatedly spoke about how she didn't feel that she had problems in common with the others, and she felt it was impossible to survive if you depended on others, because people would let you down. She continued, saying that people had brains and could make their own choices. The therapist attempted to include others, but René, with pressure of speech, talked through the intervention, stating that the medications that she was receiving were not helpful.

Ron commented that René's stories reminded him of how painful his divorce had been and the guilt he suffered. He agreed with René that people were responsible for their choices. June began talking about how someone had reported that she worked to Social Security, and she feared that this might lead to her SSDI payments being cut.

Angela then said that one could make up to $5,000 before having benefits affected. June continued to worry about whether to quit her job and how she had been victimized at the workplace. There was a continued discussion among the three "old" members about making a choice.

Angela said she was still thinking about what René had said about medication, and she did not like to take it. René described how she fooled the doctors in the hospital by spitting out her medication, and Angela added that they had wised up to her, and she received shots. She added that part of her feared stopping the shots and becoming sick and having to go back to the hospital. René then commented that if medication helped Angela, she should certainly take it.

This group, led by inexperienced clinicians, was stressed by the membership instability, and members communicated through René a sense of distrust. She responded to a therapist's efforts to interrupt her with a metaphor that the "medication" was not helpful. Ron expressed guilt, but June returned to the initial theme of distrust. Angela made her initial effort to join by providing information that was followed by a discussion conveying ambivalence about their (work) group. Angela made another effort to join by linking to experiences rejecting medication, but she also placated the doctors through acknowledging her need for treatment, which René supported by encouraging her to continue taking medication.

The therapists allowed the members to work with their feelings in the metaphor in which they powerfully communicated their distrust of others, but they also were defining how Angela was to behave. She, in turn, found a way to enter by giving advice and joining in negative feelings about her response to treatment.

Sufficient time must be provided for the group to experience and partially integrate the prospect of changes in membership. The therapist may use the opportunity to convey a number of important messages of respect for feelings and the integrity of the therapy by the manner in which new members are introduced. If the group census has rapidly diminished because of the loss of several members, a period of time must be allowed to address the feelings about the loss in the remaining members. This is never a complete process, and the actual entry of a new person will stimulate a spectrum of feelings about those who have departed.

Several scenarios are played out when the possibility of adding members is raised. Not only members but also therapists experience stress with the prospect of additions to the group. Fantasies that a newcomer will get out of control or express psychotic ideas and ruin a cohesive group are common. Embedded in these fantasies are dynamics of emotional contagion. Less evident are clinicians' anxieties that they will be recipients of induced emotions (see Chapter 10). The net result is that clinicians tend to resolve the problem by holding to the status quo, and in the process, inadvertently jeopardizing the whole group.

Review of meeting attendance may expose a downward trend that may have been denied. Because it is not always clear if a member has actually terminated or is only attending less frequently, therapists are inclined to rely on the total number of patients enrolled rather than the actual attendance as a measure of group functioning. A downward spiral of diminishing attendance, therapist discouragement, and sudden realization that the group is barely "hanging on" needs to be actively addressed and a search for new members undertaken.

The task of repopulating a group is time consuming. Optimally there are resources in which a steady flow of referrals can be counted on. Regular contact with case managers, clinic administrators, and reminders to therapists are valuable in assuring an appropriate flow of newcomers.

Therapists may decide to introduce newcomers singly or in small subgroups. The former method has the advantage of minimizing a patient's wait before joining and sets a norm in which groups can expect newcomers from time to time. The latter method, in which patients are introduced in pairs or small subgroups, has the advantage of having newcomers share the joining experience, thereby easing their entry. However, in most situations with the chronically ill population, such early identifications are not easily achieved, and the clinician must provide leadership in making linkages. If attendance has fallen to low levels, then a bolus of new members may revitalize the group, but it is preferable for therapists to replenish the numbers in a more even fashion that would not overwhelm the established patients.

Clinicians often wonder how much advance notice to provide a group that new members will be joining. The process is complicated by the structure of core and peripheral subgroups. For core members, announcements 2 or 3 weeks in advance are reasonable. This may create a situation in which more peripheral members will find a new person present with neither advance notice nor opportunity to learn about their own responses to the change. There is no easy solution to this problem, for therapists need to strike a balance between keeping patients waiting too long, extending the time for the members to process their reactions, and keeping all informed. One suggestion is the possibility of notifying the peripheral members (either by mail or phone) of the forthcoming addition(s), but such a solution may be too cumbersome to implement regularly. An alternate strategy might be to make special note of individuals who were not informed of new arrivals and actively, but not intrusively, inquire about their response to meeting another member. Even if the senior member denies or minimizes his or her response, the therapist has brought into focus an important interpersonal experience.

Overtly, most groups will not express interest in the newcomers following an announcement that others will be added to the group. There is often little direct curiosity about newcomers, with the exception of asking about gender, and discussions continue as if an announcement had not been made. Yet there is always considerable anxiety associated with the period prior to the entry, and one response may be a decreased attendance. In the discussion, associations to novel situations, unexpected family visits, or disappointments in others will likely emerge. Interpretation of these associations into the group may help the members acknowledge some of their fears and serve as an opportunity to more directly address stress. This is in keeping with the observation that reactions to anticipated or actual group boundary alterations can be addressed and integrated more easily by the members than can discussion of intermember conflicts.

> *Example*: The following vignette illustrates the intensity of one group's response to an announcement of two new individuals joining the group. Three of the four members present were diagnosed with schizophrenia. Greg, a mildly mentally retarded, passive man, worried that he might have known them from his period in a partial hospital, where people had borrowed money from him, and he had not been repaid. The therapist suggested that Greg might be concerned as well as others that newcomers might take advantage of them. Sam wondered if they were attractive women, and Jeff said he didn't like people who didn't come regularly.
>
> A theme of flight followed. Lora and Jeff discussed their efforts to find work, and Greg described his joining a new church where he felt welcomed. The therapist commented that knowing people helped in dealing with new situations, which is what they were facing. Sam worried that the room would be crowded. Jeff told of being threatened

by a group of adolescents when he was purchasing baseball tickets, a theme that became elaborated into their abhorrence of the big crowds at large city festivals. The therapist wondered if the addition of newcomers meant that the group would get too large. Jeff said there wouldn't be time for each of them.

The subsequent associations were to missing a deceased father and uncle who had provided support, and then to questions about their diagnoses and fears that they might never improve. Embedded in the discussion of their diagnosis was a sense of dehumanization. The regression was contained when the therapist suggested that members' concerns about their diagnoses suggested they would not be responded to as people with an illness, but merely as a diagnosis with little hope for change. Sam responded to this intervention at the end of the meeting by stating that if he got well, he would want to become a psychiatrist.

The intensity of the members' responses to the prospect of two newcomers supports the clinical impression that patients become intensely involved in their groups and respond with equal intensity when they fear disruption. Through understanding their fears that they would become part of a crowd and be dehumanized, the regression was reversed, as signaled by Sam's identification with the therapist.

One frequent dynamic is the fear of emotional contagion. An ever present concern of chronically ill individuals is recurrence of their major symptoms. Members express fears that hearing psychotic material will have a disorganizing effect on them. Clinicians are not immune to similar feelings. As a result, therapists have considerable reticence introducing a patient with overt symptoms of psychosis (although they may not be acutely decompensated) because they fear that the symptoms, by contagion, may infect others and destroy the group. The consequence of this process is a limitation of the candidate pool. A therapist's temptation to exclude such persons must be carefully examined for countertransferences.

Screening and Introducing the Newcomer

Proper preparation of any prospective member is essential in order to increase the likelihood of the patient remaining in the group. As discussed, in preparing members for a new group, the clinician needs to gain a reasonable diagnostic and dynamic understanding of a candidate prior to agreeing to place that person in an ongoing group. Generally, two preparatory interviews allow sufficient time to complete the tasks described in Chapter 8.

Not uncommonly, new referrals are patients who have recently been hospitalized. The staff, having observed the patient making good use of group membership in the milieu, recommend similar treatment in an outpatient setting. Under such circumstances, it may be useful to meet individually with the patients for a number of sessions to assess their degree of stability. As the length of hospital stays becomes briefer, many individuals are barely compensated when they are discharged. The stress of entering a group may overburden a precariously balanced state and lead to decompensation. Thus, a treatment plan should have sufficient flexibility to allow the clinician time to assess the patient's stability.

Adding new members to a group provides an opportunity to remind everyone of the agreement. Restatement of the basic tasks and responsibilities of membership provides a modicum of structure. It is often useful to have all present introduce themselves, but there is no requirement that anyone "tell his or her story." That information should emerge spontaneously.

Some groups will inquire about newcomers' problems, while others may overtly let the person interact in the manner they choose. Other groups may develop a norm of a go-around in which patients tell their goals. Depending on the current dynamics and the functional level of the members, new patients may be ignored. As in the example of Angela (pp. 139–140), newcomers are ignored as an expression of resentment of the intrusion, as a reaction to the therapist's "control," and as a consequence of individual problems in making social contact. However, metaphors expressing those affects (resentment, anger, ineffectiveness, and trust) emerge.

> *Example*: In a mixed racial group, one woman responded to the entry of an African American man by associating to a movie that told a story of the formation of labor union that was suffused with conflicts among the racial subgroups. This was followed by comments about a person who had lost her job and missed her work colleagues. The newcomer described his recent hospitalization and how he had trusted the nurses and doctors, and did not trust anyone else because of his illness.
>
> The following week, a veteran man talked about how his brother-in-law would come intoxicated to family gatherings and disrupt the family with threats of violence. A woman associated, "It sounds like an old movie." This was followed by further elaboration of family conflicts, warnings that violence would lead to going to jail, and that mothers did not like to take sides in fights, which was frustrating. One woman commented that her family was afraid of her when she had been sick, and that had continued even though she wasn't sick presently. The new man was then asked if he had offered a member a ride the preceding week, and he said he had not. The woman then said she would have refused it because she did not know whom she could trust.

The anxiety stimulated in this group by the entry of a new member evoked references to racial conflict, which were transformed into feelings of distrust among peers, fears of violence, and only slightly disguised outright rejection.

For some patients, the stress of entry stimulates regression, and on occasion, psychotic material will emerge. Other individuals will exhibit their stranger anxiety through excessive talking or through obvious external signs of tension, such as drumming or attention-riveting bodily movements. At times, newcomers may not be able to physically join the circle and will choose seats outside the main ring (at times, they may merely pull their chairs back). The therapist may invite them to join the circle, but patients will join in their own way and at their own pace. On occasion, newcomers will bolt from the room when their tension rises above a tolerable threshold.

The therapist may inquire if they will return, which may be a sufficient expression of interest for the departing person. Respect for the patients' "space" is indicated. Seldom is it clear if they should be pursued.

Example: Sue, a 56-year-old chronically anxious and depressed widow, was referred for evaluation by her individual therapist because of unremitting anxiety and social isolation. She had an extensive history of disabling symptoms that had not been modified with multiple medication trials or with psychotherapy. Sue was supported by pubic funds.

In the preparatory interview, Sue presented as a neatly groomed woman who barely could stop talking. She indicated that she wanted to join a group and then proceeded to tell a disconnected, rambling story in which she talked of her parents' and her husband's deaths as if they had happened within the past few months, whereas they actually had happened 4 to 10 years previously. She described the remainder of her family, including her children, siblings, and more distant relatives as unavailable and bemoaned their insensitivity to her needs. Sue was difficult to interrupt, and the therapist was aware of some frustration in attempting to do so. He was aware of some irritation in his tone as he tried to focus on some of Sue's feelings about entering a group and some of the tasks that membership entailed, including telling one's own story and being able to listen to others and provide feedback. Sue seemed able to listen to the therapist only for the briefest moments. Nevertheless, because she was motivated to enter, and discussion with the referring therapist suggested that Sue's behavior was not merely related to anticipating entering a group but had been similar to her interactions in dyadic treatment, Sue was accepted into the group. She was to continue in her dyadic treatment for several months, and then the group would be her single psychotherapeutic modality.

Sue came to the clinic for her first group meeting, neglected to register, and went to the therapist's private office. After 15 minutes, she realized her error and was directed to the group room. The members anticipating Sue's arrival had briefly inquired if she had called, but quickly shifted their interest to Kathleen's pressured story about her daughter's misbehavior. The essence of this often-repeated story was that her daughter kept promising to "turn her life around" (the daughter was heavily involved in drugs, had neglected her own children, and had walked away from a halfway house and was in violation of probation), but it had become clear to all that nothing concrete was changing. Kathleen seemed bent on trying to figure out why her daughter's behavior had not changed and was repetitively asking others why they thought her daughter was behaving as she did.

When Sue entered, the therapist briefly interrupted the story to allow for introductions and to review the group agreement. Sue, without revealing more than her name, began to interact, suggesting that Kathleen had behaved very well, and that the daughter would have to be responsible for changing. When Sue was asked if she had been in similar situations, it was as if the cork had been pulled, and a torrent of words flowed forth.

Although the others initially appeared interested and inquired about some details, they soon became restless. At that point, the therapist firmly interrupted Sue several times, directly suggesting that Sue was reacting to her experience of joining the group, and asking her to focus on those thoughts and feelings. Sue could barely acknowledge her here-and-now experience, even with several firm efforts by the therapist.

The therapist then generalized the situation, asking others to discuss their experience of entering the group. They each spoke of their memories, ranging from silent observation to anxious talking. One member then spoke of how Sue was not only anxious like others had been, but that she too was talking about how she wished her family would behave differently.

In this example, Sue's anxiety about joining a group was an additional stressor to her chronic state of anxiety. She very much wanted to belong, but the fears of again being mistreated in the group in the manner she described in her family was an added burden. The members responded to her failure to arrive on time with a lengthy discussion of irresponsible behavior, which created a less than welcoming atmosphere. Sue then presented herself in a fashion that would "test" whether she could be accepted or not. The therapist's firm intervention, stopping Sue and clarifying that part of her presentation was a reaction to the common experience of joining the group, enabled Sue to begin integration into membership. The firmness helped the others, who were showing beginning signs of discomfort and withdrawal, to reengage in the process. The structure provided by the clinician in this circumstance provides protection for all members.

Therapists need to find ways to allow new members to join in the manner in which they feel most comfortable. Among the several tasks are to recognize the stress for both old and new members, and to monitor the climate in order to prevent trauma and premature dropout. Groups will generally accept silent or withdrawn newcomers without demanding that they reveal much or any of themselves, but patients whose clinical state or anxiety leads to regression and the emergence of rambling or overtly psychotic discussion may, by contagion, have a regressive impact and lead to group fragmentation. As in the example of Sue, the clinician needs to reestablish a sense of safety for all concerned through increased activity and, if possible, accurate understanding of the process.

DROPOUTS AND TERMINATIONS

When contrasting groups for the chronically mentally ill and more typical outpatient groups, far less information is available to provide clinicians guidelines for anticipating the number of patients who will drop out either before joining the group or during the period of the initial group formation. Replacements also quit, and all must be replaced in order to maintain adequate census. In groups composed of higher functioning patients, the dropout rate for newly formed groups is in the range of 30–45% during the first 6 months (Rutan & Stone, 1993). Patients who have either concurrent dyadic treatment or have had prior therapy are more likely to remain than those who are entering a group as their initial psychotherapeutic experience. Premature termination decreases for individuals who enter into a well-formed group but may still number one-fourth of the newcomers (Stone & Rutan, 1984).

There is a far more limited body of data for groups composed of chronically mentally ill persons. It is difficult to summarize the published information, because the nature of treatment is insufficiently described and approaches vary. As a generalization, no-shows and early dropouts (within the first six sessions) ranged from 18% to 48% (Purvis & Miskimins, 1970; O'Brien et al., 1972; Herz et al., 1974). Equally variable was the reported retention rate, which ranged from 39% at 6 months to 63% at 1 year (McGee & Racusen, 1968; Herz et al., 1970; Masnick et al., 1971; O'Brien et al., 1972; Malm, 1982). A large proportion of patients in these studies were diagnosed with schizophrenia.

Review of three groups that were established utilizing the flexibly bound model in the Cincinnati program provides additional information (Stone, 1995). Attendance records were obtained for these groups from the initial session and for a period ranging from 4.5 to 6 years. Table 11.1 shows the continuers and terminators by diagnosis.

In the flexibly bound groups, 9 of 64 (14%) terminated in four or less sessions, and an additional 21 (33%) members stopped within a year. Thus, 53% remained in treatment for more than 1 year. The overall continuation rate is approximately 55%, and among the four categories, only the patients diagnosed with schizophrenia failed to continue at the 50% level.

Taking into account the limitations of the data, the rate for patients who do not appear to engage in a group (attendance of six or fewer meetings) clusters in the 20% range. Retention at 1 year varies around the 60% level. These numbers compare quite favorably with those reported with more traditional outpatient groups and suggest that chronically ill patients will attend and continue their group treatment.

Departures from the Group

Seldom are terminations in groups for chronically mentally ill planned or worked with in advance of the departure. Some patients merely disappear. They may leave the community without notification—thereby again demonstrating their fragile attachments—or they merely may decide that the group is not for them. Among the losses that are more difficult for members to manage are those persons who become medically ill, are hospitalized, and then are physically unable to return. Unexpected deaths are not rare, and the clinician's first knowledge of the death may come from group members whose community networks often are rapid sources of tragic information. It is well to remember that concurrent medical illness and problems of obtaining consistent care are well documented for the chronically mentally ill population. Members experience grief over the deceased member, and they tend to idealize the person. It may be many months later or following the departure or death of another member that negative feelings about the dead person emerge, and then in generally muted terms.

A more positive experience of termination occurs when an individual

TABLE 11.1. Continuers versus Discontinuers by Diagnosis

Diagnosis	Schiz	BiPol	UniPol	Pers & Anx	Total
Continue	7	8	5	14	34
Discontinue	11	4	4	11	30
Total	18	12	9	25	64

Note. Schiz, Schizophrenia and schizoaffective disorders; BiPol, bipolar disorder; UniPol, major depressive disorders and dysthymia; Pers & Anx, personality and anxiety disorders.

is able to secure work or enter a rehabilitation program. Often the group will be notified, but the patient may be able to attend only the meeting in which the announcement of the job is made. Full-time jobs seldom allow for time off during the day, when groups meet. Rehabilitation programs vary, but most do not provide for time to attend a therapy group. Patients who obtain part-time jobs are seldom in a position to negotiate for time off to come to therapy, and other arrangements for their continuing treatment must be made. In contrast, volunteer opportunities are more flexible, and usually patients can negotiate time to continue their treatment.

Reactions to these losses are highly variable. Individuals who only come to group for brief periods are soon forgotten, but this is not invariable. At times, members have an acute awareness of what has happened to someone who has terminated.

> *Example*: In one group, a member who had only been in the group for 3 to 4 months before she left to move to another community with her elderly mother unexpectedly walked into the group room about 8 months after she had terminated. Several members accurately recalled her last session as coinciding with Easter, and they quickly engaged her in conversation about her mother and her new living situation.

The therapist should ask patients to remain in the group for several sessions when they announce their intentions to leave. A simple explanation that the person has been a member for a period of time often will suffice, and saying good-bye is an important part of relationships. It is quite gratifying when the patient can comply with such a request.

> *Example*: Jim, a 65-year-old divorced man, had been a member for 3 years. He had been referred to group following his second arrest for indecent exposure, which he denied. His history revealed a chronic sense of loneliness, and social isolation except for frustrating contacts with one of his sons who lived with him. He was diagnosed with dysthymia, dependent personality, and exhibitionism.
>
> During his tenure in the group, Jim never revealed his arrests. He assumed an avuncular role by providing advice and support, and avoiding or dampening conflict. He seldom spoke of anything personal but gradually revealed that he was getting along better with his son. Jim was well liked; and in particular, he could tease the women in a manner that evoked smiles from them. He precipitously announced his plans to terminate from the group and ended by saying that this would be his last meeting. However, he accepted the therapist's request that he remain for four more sessions.
>
> Jim did not spontaneously address his departure during that

period. The metaphors of separation were prominent in the meetings, and the therapist would translate those into the feelings within the group. Members would then closely question Jim about his plans, what he would be doing instead of coming to the group. Their feelings of loss and wish for him to remain were intense, and the therapist was careful to separate their feelings from the decision. He reminded them that this was an autonomous decision by Jim. It was only during the final meeting that Jim, in the process of saying good-bye, brushed away tears as he took his leave.

Terminations often are not the final ending of relationships. Patients often live in the same neighborhood, attend the same church, or shop at the same grocery, and the likelihood of their meeting is considerable. Thus, they may not say good-bye in the group with an expectation that they will not meet again. This perception is reinforced by patients' extragroup contacts that develop during their treatment. Departed members live on in the group memory. Updates on the statuses of former members are intermittently a topic of discussion and serve to keep their memory alive.

SUMMARY

In this chapter, the therapist's tasks associated with maintaining the group census have been addressed. With larger total membership, the use of a flowchart serves as a simple way to maintain an overview of patients' attendance patterns. Newcomers need to be recruited and may be added singly as space is available. Groups may react intensely to prospects of new members, and they should be provided sufficient time to address their feelings and ensure that the therapist will maintain interest in them. Attention to the anxiety and the regressive potential of those who enter the group will enhance the likelihood of their successful engagement.

Dropouts and terminations are inevitable, although utilizing the flexibly bound model, patients do engage in lengthy treatment. Session census may decrease as some members move from the core to peripheral engagement. Terminations are often abrupt, but efforts should be made to help members address feelings evoked by separation.

TWELVE

SPECIAL LEADERSHIP CONSIDERATIONS

If the leader is never to oppose the will of the majority, it is difficult to see what appeal other individuals will have from the vicious fatuities to which unopposed majorities are always subject.

—SLATER (1966, p. 257)

This chapter will address a number of leadership considerations that group therapists face. The focus is on models and formats that impact upon the clinician's functioning and, by extension, influence the conduct of treatment.

Seldom is the care of the chronically mentally ill relegated to a single clinician. Indeed, multiple caregivers are involved, and group therapists become part of a team, however loosely defined. Attention to the dynamics of several of these formats can inform the clinician regarding their potential therapeutic and antitherapeutic properties.

In this chapter, dynamics of coleadership (cotherapy) and singly led models, leadership and medication, and change of therapists will be examined.

COLEADERSHIP

Most models of treatment with the chronically mentally ill suggest group leadership should be shared (Payne, 1965; Lesser & Friedmann, 1980; McGee, 1983; Stone, 1993b). There are many cogent reasons to support this recommendation and relatively few to oppose it. In contrast to higher functioning groups, most treatment takes place in clinics rather than in private-practice settings. Because treatment is conceptualized as a long-term process, optimally groups should have consistent leadership. Unfortunately, many clinics suffer staff turnover or are utilized for training sites with neophyte clinicians entering and leaving the system at regular intervals. A cotherapy model increases the likelihood of leadership continuity. Moreover, cotherapy provides an opportunity for more experienced clinicians to train neophytes, and thereby increase the pool of trained clinicians. On-the-job training with supervision is the traditional and most effective way of providing leadership training, particularly if it is combined with didactic and theoretical teaching.

Working with the chronically ill population is not an easy task, and the opportunity to share the leadership functions and to exchange ideas about the treatment process may serve as an effective antidote to the sense of uncertainty and to the frustration that is so commonplace. Certainly a number of sessions are gratifying for therapists, but the proportion of good meetings to those that are slow moving and filled with little new material is not very great. Clinicians' experiences with sharing their observations and their frustrations serve as a release and enable them to maintain their balance.

The old saying that four eyes and ears are better than two often is true, as each therapist may observe or hear different elements in the transactions. Sharing these observations broadens each clinician's understanding, and adds an element to his or her learning that diminishes the potential for burnout.

Another obvious advantage of cotherapy is the provision of continuity of leadership when one of the therapists is absent. Patients will react to the absence of a leader, and the members' feelings about absences can be usefully explored. Denial of separation does not need to be immediately challenged, but as patients emotionally invest in their therapists, the feelings of loss with even a temporary interruption may be addressed.

Some cotherapists rather slavishly try to arrange their lives so that one person is present at all sessions. It is incorrect for therapists to attempt to schedule their lives so that there is never a missed session. In practice, this would not be possible, because national and local holidays mean either canceling a meeting or trying to find an alternate day. Patients will survive an interruption caused by the absence of both therapists. Under those circumstances, therapists have made a choice not to be present. It can be a powerful message, ranging from association to abandonment to that of strength, that the patients have inner resources to manage the interruption. In our experience, patients can manage 1 or 2 weeks of not meeting. More extended periods may cause disruptions that seem to take many months to repair, and may be associated with significant decompensations.

In this respect, particular attention might be paid to the Christmas/New Year period when the holidays may disrupt the regular schedule. This time of year is often stressful, and the "myth of a happy family" may be exposed as just that. Sometimes an alternate group time between the two holidays can be found that will accommodate most members and lessen the discontinuity.

Therapists make considerable emotional investment in working with this population. They are subjected to many projections, stirring feelings of being ignored or inadequate. The parental transferences evoked by cotherapists (even if they are of the same gender) can be stressful when a clinician finds him- or herself being assigned an unfamiliar role, or a familiar role is exaggerated and a therapist becomes immobilized. The opportunity to review and process these experiences with a colleague enables clinicians to keep grounded in their work and diminishes their being derailed in a transference–countertransference stalemate.

There are obvious pitfalls in conducting cotherapy. These should not be construed to contraindicate this leadership format. Rather, alerting clinicians to some of the difficulties may prevent development of a treatment impasse or even failure.

Cotherapy is a misnomer when it is used to describe the leadership configuration of an experienced permanent staff, and a trainee, or neophyte clinician (Roller & Nelson, 1993). The newcomer is not equal to the skilled senior person in terms of understanding the patients and the group process. The differential levels may cause conflict between the leaders, which can become manifest in overt competitiveness; for example, one leader speaks immediately following the other in order to "clarify" or "add to" what has been said. In other pairs, either therapist may withdraw from a leadership position in excessive deference to the other or as a reaction to competitive strivings.

A common problem emerges in training settings in which a younger psychiatric resident is paired with a nonmedical senior staff person. Patients often will try to relate to the resident around the familiar role of physician, asking about medication changes, side effects, or prognosis. The resident, believing that a direct response is necessary in order to maintain the stance of a doctor, may answer specific questions. There is no fundamental disadvantage in responding in this fashion, and doing so may facilitate a budding therapeutic relationship. However, there is danger in role lock. The dynamic meanings underlying the questions should be assessed. For many neophyte clinicians, patients' process of asking questions is an initiation rite.

The nonmedical therapist, in the process of forming a new relationship with a physician coleader, may experience such questioning as a depreciation of his or her talents or contributions, thereby having the potential to stir conflict between the two clinicians. Attention to the timing of patients' inquiries about "medical" problems may provide a clue to their covert meaning. A variation of the medical–nonmedical split may arise when the physician is absent and the nonphysician is asked medical questions as a communication about the absent leader. Such interactions may be experienced as a put-down by the clinician who is present. Obviously, competition is not limited to therapist pairs that are unequal, but it is emphasized because it is a common treatment configuration. Patients attempt to simplify their lives by reverting to stereotypes: the doctor is to give medicine; the social worker (psychologist or nurse) is to care for patients' needs. Fuel for these splits arises in part from the clinicians' behaviors, and it behooves therapists to be aware of their own needs to feel safe in stereotypical roles.

Gender, race, and age may become a source of difficulty. Although, optimally, male–female cotherapy recreates a family constellation, patients have their own prior experiences with parents, and there may be considerable splitting and favoritism expressed toward one or the other leader. Race is a powerful stereotype. African American therapists become containers of many preconceptions that are only vaguely referred to or are addressed only in metaphor. Patients are willing to address race issues if therapists will tune in to subtle "tests." Frequently, it is therapists who have the greatest difficulty exploring issue of race between themselves or with the patients.

Of course, the leaders may have transferences to one another, stimulated by the various leadership configurations. Older sister, younger brother, controlling or passive parent or child, or more intelligent sibling are a few such relationships. Preliminary discussion between cotherapists, in which family attitudes are mutually explored, sets the stage for unconscious elements to be examined as they may emerge within the treatment process.

If the trainee remains with the group for an extended period of time (usually more than 6 months), leadership moves toward greater equality. This development may be both welcomed and serve as a stress when particular roles (e.g., the valued or "idealized" leader) are altered. Generally, such a shift is welcomed and is gratifying to the senior clinician, who has the experience of helping a colleague grow. In such a process, senior persons also learn and grow themselves.

It is essential for cotherapists to devote time and energy to their relationship. Prior to beginning work together, clinicians should spend time sharing their backgrounds and interests, and therapeutic styles and goals in working with this population. They should be clear about their commitment to one another, which would include sufficient time to process their work following each meeting. Additional time may be useful prior to the following session as each person may have used the intervening period to further integrate aspects of the therapy meeting. As in any emotionally significant relationship, change is inevitable, it is hoped, in the direction of growth. Clinicians who have successfully resolved their inevitable differences are justifiably proud of their accomplishment. The work is not only cognitive but also includes considerable exploration of each therapist's emotional responses. Both clinicians should be prepared to seek consultation in circumstances of an impasse.

One block to cotherapists' growth is a senior clinician serving as the only supervisor for the junior therapist. This arrangement has the potential for stimulating student–teacher conflicts. An additional opportunity for supervision with a third person is an antidote to some, but not all, of the potential pitfalls of this treatment–supervisory dyad.

Among the issues that need to be addressed between cotherapists are the division of administrative tasks, including starting and ending the group, dealing with their own or patient absences, record keeping, and contacts with outside agencies, family members, or case managers. These can be time-consuming tasks, and it is easy for one of the therapists to feel overburdened. Some solutions to the inevitability, at least in the short run, of unequal workloads can be counterproductive.

Cotherapists should also explore their therapeutic styles, which might include extent and content of self-revelation, openness to dealing with their in-group differences (the model of parents showing their capacity to differ), and styles of intervention to individuals, dyads, or the group as a whole. It should come as no surprise to either individual that his or her partner interacts in the group in unexpected ways. These are matters for the cotherapy team to address, usually initially in their postgroup meetings, or in supervision.

Example: A leadership misalliance followed upon the cotherapists' agreement to enter the room together. A problem arose when one of the leaders was delayed, and as a consequence, both clinicians entered the group about 10 minutes late. Several patients, who had arrived on time, had seen one therapist waiting in his office, but they did not initially acknowledge their observation. The therapists apologized for their lateness and extended the session with the agreement of the members. Fairly shortly one member told of a recent experience in which she had been waiting to catch a bus, and realized that she was hungry and had several minutes to spare before the bus was due to depart. She went to a restaurant and bought a carryout sandwich that she put in her shopping bag. There was a brief delay in making payment and another customer joined the short line at the cashiers.

The patient suddenly realized she might miss the bus and without realizing what she had done, she grabbed the second patron's sandwich. On the bus, she realized what had happened and guiltily returned to the restaurant to make restitution. The cotherapists did not understand the patient's communication about having to wait and being hungry. The basis for the cotherapists' agreement to delay until both were present before entering was addressed in supervision.

The advantages of cotherapy, particularly working with the chronically ill population, outweigh the drawbacks. Clinicians should not underestimate the difficult emotional tasks of a truly collegial relationship. Transferences frequently abound between colleagues, with expectations, hopes, and disappointments that are based both on the reality of interactions and on prior experiences. If the relationship resembles a honeymoon, there probably is a modicum of denial, because patients stimulate differences, which the clinician pair must address. Indeed, at times it seems that therapy remains at a standstill until the clinicians have effectively worked on their relationship. Despite these caveats, advantages of cotherapy accrue in the sectors of training, continuity, sharing of emotional tasks of leadership and peer learning. The "expense" of time required to attend to the therapists' relationship, however, is well rewarded if it is pursued with openness and integrity.

ALTERNATIVE LEADERSHIP MODELS

A less frequently employed leadership model is that of the single clinician. This model arises from some therapist's wish to have sole leadership, the unavailability of more than a single clinician, or from systems' decisions that the model is cost effective. Sometimes, groups begin with cotherapists and then with one person's departure, the leadership becomes solo.

The single clinician has the advantage of being able to more clearly understand certain transference configurations, such as responses to separations, deprivations, and loss in relation to his or her own specific behaviors. These feelings are most often presented in metaphor (as in the bus/restaurant example). Their translation into the here and now of the group is possible in stable groups but may be limited due to the state of the therapeutic alliance. Under these circumstances, the feelings may be productively explored in a displacement. Moreover, the single clinician does not have to attend to a cotherapy relationship. Nevertheless, the absence of a working partner should not prevent the solitary therapist from setting aside time to review notes from prior sessions. Themes or transference configurations that had escaped initial recognition sometimes emerge with striking clarity and may be invaluable in gaining an understanding of the therapeutic process (see Chapter 6 for discussion of record keeping).

In settings in which groups are singly led, a second person may assume a role of substitute therapist. This person may be available to fill in during the primary therapist's vacations or during an illness. The role may be filled by the group supervisor, or a second person may be assigned this responsibility. In some clinics, a model of alternate leadership functions to assure continuity in the absence of one leader (Levin et al., 1985). Rutan and Alonso (1980) describe a model in which leaders alternate at 3-month intervals. The individual not conducting treatment is available to observe the group with trainees behind a one-way mirror. Over extended time periods, the second (or alternate) person will develop a productive therapeutic relationship with the group.

LEADERSHIP AND MEDICATION

A large proportion of chronically mentally ill individuals receive psychotropic medications as an essential component of their treatment. Thus, it is essential for the group leader(s) to determine how each member can be assured easy, prompt, and continuing access to medication. Certainly this is not the group therapist's sole responsibility, and developing a degree of collaboration between the prescribing physician and the therapist is a shared task. However, the reality is often not so simple, unless the system is structured to simplify communication and provide patients with "user friendly" access.

Among the rapid changes taking place in the delivery of care to the mentally ill is a partial redefinition of the role of the psychiatrist. A number of authorities (Verhulst, 1991) have suggested that psychiatrists' roles may be defined within a medical model, and they will function as diagnosticians and as experts in combining psychotherapy and pharmacotherapy. Nevertheless, at this juncture there remains a degree of tension around arrangements to provide medication for patients of nonphysician caregivers (Goldberg et al., 1991; Rodenhauser & Stone, 1993). Over time, a degree of trust and respect must be nurtured in order to optimize patients' care across two therapeutic modalities for which true integration has not been conceptualized.

Three options present themselves for collaboratively providing and monitoring medication effects: (1) during the meeting, (2) at a time contiguous with the group, and (3) at a separate appointment time. In a dynamically oriented group, there are considerable drawbacks to the first option, in which prescriptions are refilled during the session. Writing prescriptions interrupts the flow of ideas, and members engage in side conversations or fall silent. In some medication groups, patients are seen in a separate office and temporarily exit the session in order to receive their medicine—an undesirable scenario. A certain degree of flexibility may be in order, because on occasion, a patient may ask to leave the meeting early. Most frequently this is caused by time conflicts arising with competing medical appointments (there are few options open to patients who make appointments in public health facilities), but it may also be linked to a family member's availability for transportation. It seems prudent to interrupt the session to manage the medication and then address others' responses as they emerge in the subsequent associations. If a pattern of early departures by either a single or multiple individuals emerges, the dynamics of the treatment require attention.

The second option has the advantage of using the medication and the group as mutual reinforcers. The medication serves as a carrot that encourages attendance at the group, particularly in the early stages when interpersonal linkages are tenuous. There are several additional advantages for providing medication immediately following the session. The group therapists have had an opportunity to assess the patient's clinical status, and they have been able to observe thinking or affective disturbances, and the presence of abnormal movements (i.e., signs of tardive dyskinesia). If the prescribing physician is also the therapist (in circumstances where he or she is the single leader, or more commonly as a psychiatric resident in a training setting), the data are already available. If medications are to be provided by another physician, the group leaders should remain during that time and openly discuss their observations regarding the patient's clinical status. This procedure ensures that the therapists are aware of any changes the prescribing physician makes with the medications, and it also serves to assure the patients that the treatment team is working collaboratively.

Some patients will tentatively join the group by arriving late or at the time medication is prescribed. The communication in such behavior is not always clear, but it may be a sign of decompensation or a reaction to events within the treatment. The others may encourage the tardy member to come on time, signaling their interest, which may have a positive effect. Withholding medication because a patient did not attend the meeting would be inappropriate.

We have found it useful to manage pharmacotherapy in the group room, rather than in a separate office. Other members may stay, and they can serve as auxiliary therapists in commenting about side effects or the necessity to continue taking medication. Two drawbacks to this arrangement are that (1) insufficient time may be allowed for a detailed review of a patient's status, and (2) when depot medication is prescribed, patients may wish to receive the injection in a private setting.

The advantages of arranging a separate time to review medications are the increased frequency of contact and the opportunity to spend sufficient time to carefully review a patient's clinical status. Expense in terms of time and actual cost are a drawback for the patient. For the clinician, this arrangement adds a layer of communication with the physician that requires care and staying power.

Because patient needs are not predictable, there are advantages for the clinician to allocate time at the meeting's end for medication and other administrative tasks. In some settings, there are requirements to formally evaluate patients for medication side effects. Administering the abnormal involuntary movement screening (AIMS) test has become a standard procedure in a number of settings. There is relatively little personal exposure for the patients in this procedure, and the AIMS test can be performed as a routine. The openness often is reassuring to patients with regard to both the quality of care and the relative innocuousness of the procedure.

The fundamental principle of collaboration among clinicians in patient care is often tested around medication. Patients can divide their loyalties and their treatment in ways that are difficult for their caregivers and for themselves. Clinicians' attention to those pitfalls will increase the likelihood of effective treatment.

> *Example*: In one group that had experienced the sudden death of a member in the preceding several months and the upsurge of suicidal ideas in another member who was unexpectedly absent, those present devoted most of the session to descriptions of disorganized and dysfunctional families. Immediately prior to the closing scheduled time, the members actively engaged the physician cotherapist in a discussion of medication side effects and efficacy. The therapist, feeling under considerable pressure, extended the meeting, much to the consternation of her cotherapist, who felt manipulated.

The therapists had the task of understanding the group process and the impact upon each of them and their relationship.

CHANGING THERAPISTS

One of the problems impacting groups for the chronically ill is changes in leadership. Leadership is transferred in a planned or unplanned fashion. Planned changes take place because full-time staff members terminate their work in the process of leaving the agency, lose interest, or experience insufficient emotional support to sustain them. Trainees come and go, and their arrivals and departures can be regularly anticipated. Unplanned transfers follow illness or death. In contrast to the private-practice sector, leadership in mental health clinics appears to change at a more rapid rate than might seem optimal for patient care. The change impacts not only patients, but also, in a coleadership situation, the remaining clinician. Good-byes and hellos are among the more significant stresses in human relationships.

The "institutional ethos" (McGee, 1980) may have a significant influence on the ease or difficulty with which transitions take place. A commitment to orderly and planful change that is organized to contain the clinicians' anxieties can ease the transition. The new therapist is likely to experience anticipatory anxieties about working with the patients and with the cotherapist. Similarly, the remaining clinician is likely having his or her own concerns about taking on a new colleague. At times in training settings, a senior clinician may tire of the stress associated with "breaking in" a neophyte and choose to terminate leadership, doubly stressing the group. The institution, through a group supervisor or consultant, will do well to be alert to emotional responses of the senior therapist and not become singularly concerned with the anxiety of the newcomer. In one setting, an annual luncheon is arranged for the senior clinicians. This acknowledges their efforts in training newcomers and, as part of the agenda, provides an opportunity to discuss each person's responses to the change.

McGee (1980) also observes that supervisors have their own responses to departing and entering therapists. The supervisor's response may impact in very important ways in easing or inhibiting successful integration of a forming therapeutic team.

Several models have been proposed to assist in the changeover: no overlap, minimal overlap, observation, and stage phasing (Rutan & Stone, 1993). These models roughly represent a continuum of increasing contact between the group and the incoming clinician. In the no overlap model, the new therapist arrives at the first scheduled meeting following the farewell of the departing therapist; in the minimal overlap model, the incoming clinician may merely come to a meeting several weeks prior to the scheduled departure and introduce him or herself, greet the members, and depart; in the observer model, the therapist may remain throughout a series of sessions in order to gain direct knowledge of the members and the process without participating except in a "socially appropriate" manner (e.g., answer brief questions, but not engage in "therapeutic" activity); and in stage phasing, the incoming clinician may first serve as a silent observer and then participate in a therapist role.

Patients who are able to manage feelings in relation to separation may well benefit from the no overlap model, because it provides the most rigorous departure and entrance. Nevertheless, two elements militate against this for the chronically ill population. First, the members' relationship with the outgoing clinician may represent one of few sustained, positive emotional experiences they have had in their lives. Parent–child relationships have often been dysfunctional, if not toxic, and the hope for an ongoing parental substitute in the person of the therapist is shattered with the departure of the clinician. The propensity for regression into severely disturbed mental states is considerable under these circumstances. Second, many of those patients have been traumatized by actual parental loss or emotional deprivation by abusive or unavailable parents. Restimulation of ambivalent feelings in anticipation of losing a surrogate (therapist) parent is often poorly handled. Therapist departures can reawaken memories of previous loss, with a mixture of feelings that include relief, shame, guilt, envy, or abandonment.

In response to change, patients may wall off feelings rather than address the loss and the associated affects. With a stage phasing model, in which the incoming therapist becomes familiar with the patients in their interaction and then assumes a more active leadership stance, there is an opportunity for the members to develop an alliance with the newcomer that will sustain them through the stress of a changeover.

The clinical management of the transfer and the feelings evoked in the departing therapist are often difficult. If a trainee knows that he or she will be with the group for a designated period, this may be announced at the beginning. However, patients seldom "remember" this information and will inquire if the trainee is going to depart. Of course, they hope that the original information is false. Exploration of the feelings should proceed slowly, and generally a question can be responded to with a direct reality answer ("I will be leaving the clinic on June 18"). Patients will respond to the information in their own characteristic fashion, and little is achieved by inquiring into members' feelings or fantasies before answering. In groups that have had a series of trainees as leaders, patients anticipate the annual change, and often at a midyear point the question arises whether the therapist will continue beyond the end of the academic year.

> *Example*: One specially difficult change occurred with the loss of the permanent staff member, who had led the group for 7 years, the resident cotherapist, and unavailability of new therapists. A plan was developed to merge two groups. Four months in advance of the change, both therapists announced that they would be leaving. The resident's announcement was a reiteration of what he had announced at the beginning of his tenure, but the staff member's announcement was a shock, and almost all of the initial attention was directed at her departure. Chuck said that he would miss her. Miriam asked why she was leaving, and she was told that it was a career change. Chuck said it was time for him to leave, and he would prefer an individual therapist. Greg said that he belonged to two support groups, and he

did not need to continue; he only wanted to arrange for his medication. Miriam told how her adolescent son had run away again and was unmanageable, so she had given up on him. Chuck said that the restaurant that he was working at had gone to hell; the cook had been arrested for drug abuse, waiters had quit, and the manager was not effective in holding the place together.

The metaphors were very clear to the therapists who began their work knowing that they had a difficult 4 months ahead. They directed the discussion back into the group and were able to assist the patients in exploring their feelings of disappointment, hurt, loss, helplessness, anger, and flight. The staff member, who had experienced patients' reactions to changeover of four previous residents, remarked that she was keenly aware of her own inner reactions to having to tell the group of her departure. She had commented to a colleague prior to her announcement that the patients would not be able to talk about her leaving. In the session, she was initially flooded with sadness and guilt as she heard the associations, and for a time was immobilized before she could begin to helpfully intervene.

> *Example*: In another group, the pregnant resident announced that she would be leaving at the end of the academic year, 3 months hence. A member asked if she was going to stay home and be a mother or continue to work as a psychiatrist. The therapist was startled because, although she was in the early part of the second trimester of her first pregnancy, she had not told the members that she was pregnant. She told them that her plans were to care for her baby and then return to work. The subject was overtly dropped, but within a few minutes the members began to discuss relatives or acquaintances whose infant children had died suddenly in their crib (sudden infant death syndrome [SIDS]). One member, who had participated in the discussion of SIDS and whose relative had experienced such a death, commented to the therapist that the baby had looked like her.

In this example, archaic envy of the baby and destructive rage at the therapist dominated the group atmosphere. The members felt abandoned and jealous of the unborn baby receiving the therapist's attention, and in their rage they wished to destroy the offending objects (therapist–mother and infant). The therapist, understanding the process, was able to contain her own feelings and listened respectfully. The cotherapist was able to begin a more direct discussion of feelings related to loss.

> *Example*: In another group suffused with intense feelings aroused by a change in therapists, a 42-year-old schizophrenic man, when he heard that the staff woman therapist was leaving, quit his job that he had held for several years. He explained that when he drove to work,

he passed a street that had the same name as the only woman that he had ever made love to, and he could no longer tolerate seeing her name each day. He found another job, which threatened his ability to regularly attend meetings. Fortunately, he quickly became dissatisfied with the new position, and as feelings of loss were addressed, he decided to return to his old job and remain in the group.

These examples belie the notion that chronically ill patients do not form intense attachments in their therapy. Indeed, the opposite is often true. The therapeutic challenge is to manage patients' feelings so that they may become integrated into their psychic structure and do not lead to destructive responses to self or other. In the context of patients' tendencies to experience their reactions of anger, rage, or envy to the threatened separations as dangerous or disorganizing, considerable sensitivity is required. These emotions can be examined initially in terms of loss and aloneness, and later the destructive affects can be addressed more directly.

Over a period of time, patients do begin to manage their feelings over separation. The man who changed jobs had dealt with resident departures during the first 4 years he was in the group by leaving the community for a period of 3 months, so that he would not experience the transition. Thus "merely" changing jobs and not leaving the community was a considerable accomplishment.

SUMMARY

In this chapter, common leadership issues have been reviewed. Cotherapy is the most common treatment model, but it requires care and nurturing in order to optimize effectiveness. In situations in which cotherapy is not employed, arrangements for a substitute or an alternating clinician minimize disruptions. Provisions for medication are essential in any work with this population. If the group is led by a nonphysician, arrangements should be made for the person monitoring medication to meet jointly with the therapists and the patient, optimally, immediately following the close of the session.

Groups for chronically ill persons often involve trainees who depart at regular intervals. Staff members also are prone to burnout and depart from leadership. Clinicians should not underestimate the intensity of members' engagement with their therapists, and they should provide sufficient time to assist in the transition process.

THIRTEEN

SPECIAL TREATMENT CONSIDERATIONS

In dealing with people, one must realize that there are always reservations in communication—things that all of us are taught from the cradle onward as dangerous to even think about, much less to communicate freely about.

—SULLIVAN (1970, p. 206)

In this chapter I will consider elements of the treatment process that emerge in working with chronically ill individuals. Not all topics can be addressed; some situations occur with sufficient frequency to impact upon the treatment process and thereby provide opportunities for both gain or deterioration.

MEDICATIONS

Arrangements for providing patients their medication were described in Chapter 8, and medications and cotherapists were described in Chapter 12. In this section the metaphorical and communicational aspects of patients' discussions of medicines will be examined in greater detail.

Multiple levels of communication are activated when a person inquires about medication. Communication is further expanded when other members contribute to the discussion, although a single individual may serve as a spokesperson and convey important "information" for the entire group. The surface level of an inquiry or question is frequently overt and practical. A person may request information: "Does the medication

I'm taking cause such and such side effects?" "Can I reduce my medication?" "Will these medications become habit forming?" "Can I get something for sleep?" "Is there a medication that will be helpful for my symptoms?" Other levels are covert, and they are usually associated with an affective response within the clinician. The therapist's reaction is a response to a "message" regarding an emotional state of a particular individual, the group as a whole, or the treatment environment. Zaslav and Kalb (1989) suggest that discussion of medications carries hopes and fears about treatment and personal progress, self-efficacy, and attitudes about control and authority. A clinician thus must determine which level requires the most attention and the potential meaning for the members in choosing one or another level.

These are not easy choices. Responding to the direct request for information may provide useful information but close off exploration of covert meanings. Poorly timed exploration of preconscious or unconscious meanings may be experienced as a narcissistic injury and disrupt a fragile treatment alliance. Unfortunately, there is no formula prescribing a proper intervention that will serve to allay a clinician's uncertainties.

Medications and the Therapist

Often patients introduce medications into the discussion as a vehicle to convey negative feelings about the therapist. They may feel neglected, mistreated, or injured in a variety a ways, which they communicate with questions about the specific benefits of a medicine, discussion of discomfiting side effects, or overall efficacy of drug treatment. Patients experience an injury, either consciously or unconsciously, and "choose" to talk about their medicines as a way of conveying their injury ("bad side effects") or their disparagement of the therapist ("Medicines the doctor gave me don't help"). A sudden shift to the positive effects of pharmacotherapy may convey similar emotions; the message is that medicine is better than group treatment. A frequent stimulus leading to talk about drugs is an interruption in the regular treatment schedule due to a therapist's absence or a holiday. The change stimulates feelings of loss and abandonment, which are metaphorically addressed through the medium of medicine. Members may react similarly to other changes, such as introduction of a new member or another person's decompensation requiring hospitalization. Of course, misunderstandings or conflict with the therapist can be experienced as threatening, and a patient may request medication as an effort to be soothed. Medicines also represent control. Patients can choose to take their drugs or not, which serves as an antidote to helplessness.

Not all discussions of medication carry negative messages. Some patients introduce medications into the discussion as a way of clarifying aspects of their relationship with the group leader. Patients who have missed a number of sessions may return to the group and reintroduce themselves by indicating that they had altered their medication in some fashion. This may be an attempt to engage their therapist in a test to determine how they will be accepted. The reentry phenomenon may hide shame or guilt in relation to the absence(s), and patients often seek reassurance of acceptance before they tell of emotional significant reasons for their absence. In this context, then, it is unnecessary for the clinician to be the prescribing physician in order for a patient to utilize this avenue of reentry. An abrupt dismissal of the patient's communication or a comment that medications can be discussed at "a more appropriate time" can be deleterious to the treatment relationship.

In groups co-led by a physician and nonphysician, the nonmedical person may be harangued with questions about medication during the colleague's absence. Many nonphysician clinicians experience such discussion as a disparagement of their psychological work and thereby miss the opportunity to search for other meanings. The discussion can convey the members feelings about loss and contain a challenge for the remaining therapist to help contain and work with their reaction to separation.

Many therapists, including physicians, although recognizing that some individuals will need medication for the duration of their lives, view pharmacotherapy with ambivalence. A therapist may be very comfortable maintaining a schizophrenic patient on antipsychotic medication, but when a patient requests anxiolytic or sedative/hypnotic drugs, the therapist may express some reservations about the wisdom of the request. This reaction potentially communicates a clinician's negative attitude. In the thrall of a negative transference, exploration of the patient's reasons for asking may be perceived by the patient as a refusal, which adds to the disruption of the treatment alliance.

Patients may insistently communicate their need for medication. It is difficult under intense emotional pressure to determine if the medication can be therapeutically beneficial or if "giving in" is a countertransference enactment. Thus a clinician's discomfort can be used as an opportunity for self-exploration and examination of countertransference.

Medications and the Patient

Patients' self-esteem is often closely linked with their feelings about medication. Patients may attribute negative self-images to their pharmacotherapy. Dynamic considerations leading to patients rejecting medicine include their view that medication is evidence of their continuing illness, their power struggles with the therapist (and with other members), their desire for personal efficacy, or their competitive strivings with other members. Among the positive dynamic configurations are responses that medicines serve as a stabilizing transitional object (Adelman, 1985), or that they have helped in gaining control over thought or mood disorders. In a number of circumstances, the wish for the therapist's attention (dependency or narcissistic needs) is paramount.

> *Example*: Ms. A began the group by describing a fall at the grocery store that resulted in contusions and "problems with her head." One therapist showed considerable concern and made a number of inquiries about her physical and emotional state. Mr. B, diagnosed with schizophrenia, turned to the physician cotherapist and inquired about medications he had been receiving. Unfortunately, the cotherapist told him that this would be discussed at the end of the session. Mr. B became silent, and when he eventually spoke, he said that he was doing well, implying little need for the group. The therapist had not "heard" the competitive request for attention.

Medication may be introduced into a discussion as a method of regulating interpersonal distance. Intimacy often is a frightening experience for seriously ill patients, and when a sense of too great closeness emerges or a particularly intimate exchange has taken place, patients may attempt to regain their balance by shifting the discussion to medication.

> *Example*: A group discussion focused on gains that members (diagnosed with schizophrenia or schizoaffective disorder) had made over the prior 3 to 4 years. Ms. M was working steadily 25 hours a week at her first sustained job in 17 years; Mr. N had begun to develop some social relationships that were not intimate, but had some reality basis (i.e., he would go out to lunch or play tennis with women he met at his volunteer job); Mr. O was working with a case manager to enter a rehabilitation program, and Ms. P was discussing how she had changed in the group from a monopolizer to being able to listen, which pleased her and the others. As this discussion continued, Mr. N said that none of the changes he made would have been possible without his private doctor prescribing the proper medication. The experience was of devaluation of the group and Mr. N's distancing himself from the others.

As in this example, patients may introduce a discussion of medication to alter the therapeutic process and try to regain a sense of balance when there have been "unmanageable" disturbances in their relationships with others or with the group as a whole (Rodenhauser & Stone, 1993).

Certainly one benefit of group membership is an ability to be helpful to others. Medications may be an avenue of making contact as patients share benefits and difficulties with taking their drugs. It is not unusual for patients to strongly support continuing their medicines when someone is decompensating. Peer support is a powerful tool and can evoke a sense of considerable self-efficacy (Rodenhauser, 1989).

Medications and the Treatment Environment

In many circumstances the treating therapist does not provide medication. The physician who does may communicate negative attitudes about either the medicine or the role requirement of collaboration with nonmedical personnel (Goldberg et al., 1991). Patients perceiving the prescriber's attitude then may act on conflicts between their clinicians by depreciating or altering how they relate to their medicine or to the group.

Events in a clinic setting may be brought into the group room and discussed through the medium of medicine. In one situation, a psychiatrist who had been providing medications abruptly departed from the clinic, and feelings about his departure were initially communicated in terms of medicine. Other circumstances in the extragroup setting specifically linked to medications are delays in obtaining results of laboratory tests or mix-ups in arrangements for obtaining necessary testing. These impact upon patients' treatment and understandably are brought into the group.

Medications are powerful therapeutic agents because they alter neurochemistry, but they also have personal meaning to each individual. Clinicians can provide important communication channels as they work to integrate both biological and psychological messages in patients' discussion of their medications.

DREAMS

The clinical use of dreams in groups of chronically mentally ill does not assume the importance that it might in groups of less impaired individuals. This does not stem from changes in dreaming associated with chronic mental illness. Sleep studies have not demonstrated differences in dream (rapid eye movement [REM]) time between schizophrenic patients and normal controls (Dement, 1955; Feinberg et al., 1964). Depressed patients take longer to fall asleep, awaken during the night, and their REM time may be decreased, although it is subject to rebound (Hawkins, 1970). Dream content of schizophrenic individuals may be more hostile, more affective, and contain more evidence of thought disorder than those of nonschizophrenic persons (Kramer & Roth, 1979). Nightmares are not thought to be indicative of a specific diagnoses (Davis, 1967).

The apparent paucity of patients reporting dreams may be a result of interactions among members, with the therapist, or the group as a whole.

Patients know that clinicians are interested in dreams, and they may report them in hopes of gaining relief from disturbing dreams, obtaining help with symptoms of their illness, or receiving attention. They may not recall dreams or, if they do, choose not to report them because of frightening content and fears that discussion may stir unmanageable affects. Moreover, if the therapist consistently chooses to ignore dreams, patients will also stop presenting them.

It is useful to consider all dreams (perhaps with the exception of those of patients suffering from posttraumatic stress disorder [PTSD]) as a commentary about the treatment. Taking such a position does not mean that the therapist necessarily makes an interpretation or directly explores the transference implications of a dream. By thinking of dreams as a communication about the treatment, therapists might gain an understanding of the individual or perceptions of the group that had previously been obscure.

Certain themes or images appear in the manifest dream content that reflect common aspects of the treatment experience. Dreams of crowds or of strangers, often with associated anxiety are barely disguised representations of the group situation. Travel dreams generally represent treatment—the patient is going somewhere. These dreams may reflect several aspects of the treatment. Is the mode of transportation safe? Who is in charge? Is the driver or pilot qualified? Are the passengers unruly, kind, or hostile? Is the road safe or unmarked? In other dreams, unidentifiable individuals may be involved in acts of violence or destruction. The "unidentified" person may represent aspects of the dreamer or fears evoked in the treatment, either of the dreamer's own impulses or those of others.

> *Example*: With only a few minutes of the session remaining, Karen reported a dream from the preceding evening. She dreamt that she was in her apartment, and somebody brought in a casket. She knew the casket contained her deceased ex-boyfriend, who she thought was a Mafia member. She wanted the casket removed from her home. Karen associated to her boyfriend, who she felt had treated her well, but he had not revealed what he did for a living. She believed it was an illegal occupation. Karen had no additional thoughts about the dream, nor did any of the members.

The paucity of associations and the brevity of time limited the work that could be done with the dream. The therapist assumed that the casket and the Mafia member represented aspects of Karen that she wished did not exist inside her. The image evoked scenes of violence and murder for the therapist, and Karen's association to her boyfriend not revealing his profession was a communication of her own reluctance to explore more of the meaning. The discussion prior to the dream report had been of resentment of doctors. In the context of when the dream was told, one possibility was that it represented a disguised expression of resentment about the therapist. Even more speculatively, members understood this communication, and like Karen, chose not to directly express hostility to the therapist as they had toward other caretakers.

The clinician can look for the affect(s), which are often the least disguised dream elements, as an opening to understanding the dream's meaning(s). Rather than interpreting the dream in direct relation to the group, considerable therapeutic work can be accomplished by remaining in the metaphorical dream language. This strategy may be less threatening to the members by providing emotional distance. For example, in the dream reported by Karen, the therapist might have wondered aloud if the dream was an expression of her wish to free herself from difficult feelings related to her boyfriend or to illegal acts. The thought could be generalized that perhaps Karen would not be alone with such wishes. Even if this were not exact, it would demonstrate an interest in the dream and explore a theme. The therapist then might link the difficult feelings to what they had been talking about in relation to being angry with physicians, and how uncomfortable that is when patients need the doctors to care for them.

Dreams are reported in the continuing context of treatment. Even the circumstance in which a patient begins a session with a dream likely communicates feelings about a previous session. The more usual situation in which a dream is told during the meeting may be a commentary about the treatment process, and the prior discussion can be viewed as associations to the dream.

> *Example*: Steve, a newcomer to the group, was one of three men present with a male therapist. Steve and Will were diagnosed with paranoid schizophrenia; Gene was diagnosed a dependent personality. Following a beginning segment in which the members discussed the value of taking their medication, the discussion turned to Steve, who recalled having been mugged while walking in a "dangerous neighborhood." This led to a series of associations about uncontrolled teenagers acting up on buses or skipping school, and violence in movies (Steve said he didn't like to watch movies because they gave him nightmares), and then to the greater danger of guns and knives, and continued on into the need to avoid certain neighborhoods.
>
> The therapist then commented, "It is so important to feel safe. I think people worry about that as much as anything, that they can get physically attacked, that something will happen to them." Steve then asked what causes nightmares. The therapist responded that it was a form of dreaming, and everyone dreams. Steve then reported a dream:

"I was in the army; I was never in the army or in the service. I was trying to save this guy in the nightmare. I started running away, and they shot me in the back. I woke up screaming." When the therapist inquired about the buddy, Steve added, "He was running away from them too. They shot him in the leg. I was trying to pick him up, and they shot me in the back."

Steve asked what the dream meant, and Gene said that he had a nightmare, too, of "some guy coming after him." Steve told about a phone call he had received in which a man threatened to kill him. He continued, stating that recently he had been hallucinating frightening and threatening voices. The therapist wondered if there had been something that had set the dream off, and Will asked if Steve had been watching movies. After a pause, Steve recalled a movie he had been watching in which a father was beating his children. Steve said he would buy a gun to protect himself, but his brother, who lived in the home, was schizophrenic and he didn't want to have a weapon. He then added, "One thing I can say about my father, he was protective you know; he was protective about us." Will, however, continued with the theme, recalling a newspaper story in which a mother had shot her infant son in the stomach. The meeting ended on this note.

Steve's dream was reported in a context in which a question of the value of group treatment was expressed in a medication metaphor. This was followed by a discussion of violence. The therapist's intervention on the universal need for safety was framed in terms of physical safety, and the evident transference meaning of the emotional safety linked to the arrival of a new member was not directly addressed. However, the therapist had communicated his attunement to the discussion.

The dream represented a further elaboration of Steve's internally based fears. Gene's report of a dream fragment linked him with Steve, who then associated to his hallucinations, which emphasized the intrapsychic aspect of his concerns. Manifestly, the dream also conveyed Steve's efforts to help a colleague, which may have set the stage for the help that he received from the others. The therapist's efforts to explore a precipitant for the dream was responded to by introducing the topic of movies, which enabled members to continue the discussion at an emotionally manageable distance. They did not ignore or suppress the dream, but worked with it. The members' perceptions of the therapist were alluded to in references to what parents did to children. Steve's positive perspective of his father was insufficient to soothe Will, who countered with a story of a mother shooting her child. The group's ability to work with this degree of violence and aggression does not occur frequently, but it illustrates patients' capacities to explore difficult and threatening themes.

PERIPHERAL MEMBERS

The traditional emphasis on group cohesion is altered when the structure of the flexibly bound model is introduced. No longer is each absence explored and questioned. Instead, dynamics of a less tightly knit organization emerge.

Patients who attend on a regular schedule of once every 2–3 weeks seem to be fairly readily integrated into the fabric of the group. Those who attend less frequently may be greeted as if they belonged to the core group, or they may be politely greeted and then ignored. Some peripheral individuals will become assertive and quickly participate in the discussion, and others will sit back and remain peripheral.

> *Example*: Angie, a group member for 16 years, suffered several major delusional depressions prior to her referral to group treatment. She was maintained on antipsychotic and antidepressant medications, and had been rehospitalized only once during her group treatment. Initially she attended weekly and then regularly but less frequently, until she reached a bimonthly schedule. Angie always calls to learn if the therapist will be present on the week she plans to attend.
>
> Angie participates actively when present. She particularly greets senior members as if they were old friends. They, in turn, are pleased to see her. Angie makes efforts to tell newcomers a bit about herself. The group provides her with continuity, support, and a place to receive and monitor her medication in a very cost-effective and therapeutically enduring manner.

Angie represents a subgroup of patients who utilize the group in this manner. Having stabilized their illness, they engage in the group relationships in a limited but sustaining fashion.

On occasion, members may question individuals who intermittently appear, inquiring if they could attend more often. Their usual responses put members off with a series of reasons that they are unable to attend. As with other resistances, patients are unlikely to directly reveal the dynamic reasons for their attendance patterns. Some patients only minimally engage in the treatment as an enactment of their interpersonal needs and capacities. Others, like Angie, alter the relationship to the group as their condition stabilizes and do not "need" the group as they did earlier in the course of their illness. Still others seem to enter the core subgroup, and in response to the treatment process, may either terminate or move to a peripheral subgroup.

The clinician can explore the reactions of patients who appear to pressure others to attend more regularly. Ostensibly all patients have agreed to the group structure, and by not "accepting" that element in the agreement, they are exposing an aspect of themselves. Considerable tact is required in approaching these interactions. The therapist does not want to convey criticism of the patient for expressing a wish for greater involvement.

The flexibly bound model has the potential for evoking clinicians' countertransference responses. Therapeutic ambition, with the hope of helping patients participate more fully in the group, may interfere with therapists' capacity to manage their own responses to patients who attend intermittently. Countertransference reactions seem more difficult to contain when patients do not fulfill their agreement, even if that is to attend biweekly or monthly. In the circumstances in which peripheral, intermittent members participate seemingly very comfortably when they do attend and yet are suffering serious difficulties in their lives, therapists are more likely to excessively pressure them to increase their attendance.

> *Example*: In one ill-conceived response to patients' irregular attendance, the therapist sent a notice to members, stating that if patients did not attend the group twice monthly, they could not receive their medication from the clinic. Needless to say, not only were there terminations, but members also produced associations to control and Nazi atrocities.

DIFFICULT CLINICAL SITUATIONS

There are many clinical situations that perplex clinicians. We have no satisfactory taxonomy, but these situations often involve an individual apparently grossly interfering with group developmental processes. Although the focus of difficult situations appears to be on an individual or subgroup, it is important to consider the group-as-a-whole perspective as well. In this category of monopolizing–masochistic patients, complications of outside contacts, responses to death, and acting out will be discussed.

The Monopolizing Masochist

Among the more problematic clinical situations are patients who enact demands for attention and demonstrate attendant self-absorption and insensitivity to the presence of others. Such individuals repetitiously describe events in which they have been abused or mistreated and engage others in efforts to solve unsolvable external problems. Of course, others' suggestions are given short shrift, either by indicating that they have been tried and failed or, more simply by being ignored.

From an interpersonal perspective, these individuals' control of meetings serves to protect them from emotionally engaging in a relationship that they fear will be injurious. Another perspective is that of turning passive into active, a dynamic process in which individuals subject others to the experiences they have had in the past, in the hope that they may learn new ways of managing their emotions (Weiss, 1993).

From a group dynamics perspective, monopolizing masochists may arise and fill a group role that protects others from revealing themselves. The group function is revealed when the masochistic individual is absent and others fall silent or another person is "called upon" to fill the role. Nevertheless, members' manner of participation reveals important information about their own dynamics.

One dynamic is exposed in a common sequence in which members offer helpful suggestions or advice. Eventually they become weary when the monopolizer is unable to make use of their help. They may then grill the monopolizer, blaming him or her for being passive and allowing repeated abuse. This aggression represents members' efforts to address their own experiences of feeling passive, controlled, and/or abused. From this perspective, members are acting as if they do not have similar emotional responses, and their questioning serves as an emotional release and method of silencing the offending person. The monopolizer thus becomes a recipient of "justifiably" sadistic attacks, and in the group process has enacted a masochistic position. These interactions may eventuate in the monopolizer cum masochist either becoming peripheral or altogether stopping treatment.

A less malignant dynamic resonates for members with the content of a masochistic person's stories that resemble similar experiences in chronically ill individuals' lives. As a consequence of their illness and concomitant diminished social skills, the others have suffered in similar ways, and they too are at a loss as to how to extricate themselves from abusive situations. The monopolizer role thereby serves to demonstrate their helplessness. Thus, the role also contains a wish for the therapist to provide a magical solution.

The frustration of working with these individuals and their impact upon the entire group is very difficult to manage.

Example: Alex was chronically anxious and dependent. He received disability for his emotional problems, in addition to physical ailments that prevented him from working. In the group he repetitiously monopolized sessions, describing how family members from another state would visit, run up his long-distance phone bill, eat meals without paying (he also bought them special foods), and not even clean up after themselves. His sister would generally give him small amounts of money following each visit. Members initially tried to provide advice, which failed, and then they would become angry with Alex for his passivity. He would respond that he was praying that a legal judgment from a car accident would be made in his favor so he could pay his bills, and then he wouldn't put up with them. The incongruity of this solution was not lost on the members, because his debts increased with every visit.

In the evolving treatment process, members seemed to merely listen and wait until Alex finished before discussing their problems, but simultaneously they experienced a sense of helplessness. The clinician's interpretations addressing passivity were followed by associations to hopelessness and failure by the members. The therapist's efforts to help address Alex's underlying fears of loneliness and feelings of inadequacy that led him to trade his relatives visits for a bit of interest in him were of little help. Alex's attendance pattern shifted from that of a core to a peripheral member status.

In this vignette Alex demonstrated quite directly his needs for attention and his continuing wish for a magical cure. Asking Alex to listen to others was only temporarily successful, and if the therapist became too firm, Alex would miss a series of meetings. Members initially were interested, but then became bored with Alex, and the group deteriorated into an alternating sado–masochistic experience for all.

Several paths are available for the therapist to address this group issue. One possibility, described in the example, is to ask the patient to refrain from continuing to tell stories of abuse, and to provide space for others to respond. This intervention, in part, protects the members from excessive intrusion and frustration that might endanger group functioning, but it also raises the specter that others might be cut off when they are talking about important experiences. At times, despite this concern, the best strategy is for the therapist to intervene and stop the monopolizing person.

Another possibility is to focus on members' feelings of helplessness. This latter strategy, which both identifies a theme and addresses affects, may shift group interaction from one of passivity to members beginning to examine how they have handled situations in which they have been abused. This process optimally might eventuate in taking pressure off of the monopolizer (members are reowning their projections) and removing him or her from an isolated, scapegoat position. The interaction then shifts from one of advice giving or sadistic attacks to one of focusing on each individual's responsibility in his or her own fate.

Therapists can utilize their countertransference response to monitor the state of the group. Feelings of frustration, boredom, irritation, and passivity ("Let the members stop him; it is their group") are commonplace and reflect some or all of the central affects experienced by members.

Masochistic monopolizers seldom alter their emotional position following one or two interventions. The difficulty in changing these patterns is considerable. One only has to think of how difficult it is for spouses to leave their abusing partners to appreciate this difficulty. Nevertheless, some individuals do respond and change, generally over protracted periods. Often in retrospect, the clinician realizes the "offending" person is different.

The Scapegoat

As described in Chapter 5, the scapegoat is representative of the deviant-member role. These are persons who, through personal characteristics sometimes outside awareness, invite rejection from others for particular characteristics that are "unacceptable" to the others. The scapegoat engenders hostility from others, but the basis for the feelings includes mixtures of conscious and unconscious elements, and through emotional contagion, an entire group may be involved in the scapegoating process (Scheidlinger, 1982).

The dynamics of scapegoating are conceptualized in the frame of projective identification, in which aspects of the projector are "placed" into a recipient. In turn the projector identifies with the recipient (Horwitz, 1983). Although much easier described than accomplished in the therapeutic encounter, the treatment task centers around helping group members recognize in themselves the feelings that they have deposited into the scapegoat.

Elements of scapegoating are present in the group interaction with the monopolizing masochist. The exhibitionism of the monopolizer touches on each person's (unacceptable) wish to be the center of attention. Thus a portion of the hostility and ostracism that such members engender is a dynamic product of others not wishing to face their own greedy needs for attention.

Many behaviors may serve as stimuli for scapegoating. Absences or erratic attendance may stimulate others' wishes to flee the treatment setting, and consequently they reject members who do not conform. In some situations, members will challenge an ill colleague. The presence of delusions may serve as a stimulus, particularly when others are also uncertain about their own psychic equilibrium.

> *Example*: Sheldon often mentioned that he had been married and had a number of children. However, any question asking for names or dates was deflected, raising questions in members' minds if what he said was true. He also talked about feats during his military service that were more patently delusional. Thomas, who suffered a recent

rejection by a woman, began challenging Sheldon about his wife and then about his wartime experiences. Thomas seemed bent on "showing up" Sheldon, who in response to the questions became progressively grandiose and delusional. The therapist, too late, directed Thomas to desist. Within 2 weeks Sheldon terminated from the group.

The scapegoating and extrusion of Sheldon was not merely a product of Thomas's interrogation, but included the passive acquiescence of the others, who identified with the "attack," presumably as the unacceptable, grandiose delusions emerged.

The therapist also gained a more complete understanding of Sheldon's vulnerability, and as a result was able to respond more effectively when Sheldon asked to join another group.

> *Example*: On one occasion when the discussion of shame over having to ask for assistance to go shopping emerged, Sheldon grandiosely claimed to own banks, airplanes, and several cars, and thus he could travel at will. The therapist, alerted to the potential for scapegoating, was able to help members see that Sheldon was expressing some of their own desires. Sheldon was then able to interact in the session within the context of the discussion.

Therapists also can stimulate the group to search for a scapegoat. Under circumstances in which the clinician has not accurately understood the treatment process, members may turn on a peer who is labeled as insensitive and misunderstanding. If a member is suddenly criticized or becomes the object of attack, the therapist may find the basis for these behaviors in his or her own group interaction. Such displacements are more likely to occur when the therapist becomes focused on "trying to make a point," or insisting that members examine certain processes.

Scapegoating is a frequent process, and as with many situations, it presents an opportunity for members to learn about themselves. Attention to the projective elements does not imply that those aspects in the scapegoat that stimulated others are neglected. However, under circumstances in which patients have limited capacity to examine their own feelings, accomplishing these tasks is problematic. Thus it may be necessary for the clinician to firmly stop scapegoating interactions and protect the recipient prior to gaining a clear appreciation of the involved dynamics.

Complications of Outside Contacts

Extragroup contacts among members are frequent, and in most circumstances provide patients additions to their limited social networks. The tendency for such contacts to create subgroups is considerable, and characteristic of such subgroupings is a proclivity to make them special and not share their existence. References to the presence of extragroup contacts emerge under many circumstances, but patients frequently reveal their presence when a member is absent or ill and someone will provide a detailed explanations for the absence: A member might be hospitalized for medical reasons, a relative in another state has died and he or she left the city, or baby-sitting obligations arose. The information might be secondhand, as the patient had been called first by another member. These revelations generally are received positively, and the sense of exclusion is not addressed.

On occasion patients' relationships outside of the group turn sour. Members contacts between sessions reflect their interpersonal difficulties, and they may evolve into one person making demands for time, attention, and sometimes for money. In part these complications arise from the "offending" individual's unawareness of the interpersonal implications of the behavior.

> *Example*: A schizophrenic man whose wife had recently divorced him was flirtatious and made numerous comments with sexual overtones in the meetings. Outside of the group, he pursued several of the women, who had considerable difficulty preventing him from contacting them. One changed her phone number. Another, following several heated confrontations in the sessions, terminated from the group.

> *Example*: In another group, a schizophrenic woman, who frequently was in conflict with her family, would call group members late into the evening and, at times, after midnight. She seemed unable to contain her anxiety or the calls, and her family conflicts became enacted in the group. The therapist told her the calls would have to stop and that she could contact the psychiatric emergency service if she needed to talk.

It is unusual for members to become sexually involved with each other, although some personality-disordered patients seem almost preordained to locate prospective vulnerable objects for their sexual urges. More frequently, the contacts seem to be in the service of managing anxiety or trying to manage loneliness or dependency needs. Sometimes the extragroup contacts provide an opportunity for a corrective emotional experience, one that differs markedly from those of the family of origin.

> *Example*: Claire was a volatile patient, diagnosed with borderline personality disorder. She had recently returned to the group after a 2-year hiatus. Her return had been rocky, as old members recalled her

emotional outbursts and her erratic behavior, which had frightened and angered them. Group attendance diminished as several regular members began missing meetings. Following a meeting, Claire arranged with Warren, a member, to phone her at a specified time, but then she was not home to receive the call.

The succeeding session began with a muted disagreement initiated by Claire about the room being too hot. She would get up go to the window, remain for a moment, and then return to her seat. She then said to Warren that he sounded angry on her answering machine, an accusation that he denied. Dorothy said she didn't like hearing their ensuing disagreement. The senior therapist responded that she thought it was important to talk this out. Warren continued, saying that it was "no big deal." Claire again got up and stood behind Warren by the window.

Dorothy then "observed" that she, Warren, and the therapist each had a big stomach. The therapist, startled, wondered if Dorothy changed the topic because she had become uncomfortable. This led Dorothy to discuss the violence in her own family, including a recent episode in which she had been choked. The cotherapist then commented that she thought both Warren and Claire had wished Claire had been home, which meant they had similar wishes. Both protagonists agreed, and Dorothy added that for Easter she would not return home, where she would be subjected to family fighting. Instead, she would go to the Day Treatment Center where she could enjoy a meal.

In this session the therapist acted firmly to contain the anger over the disappointments involved in a botched outside contact. With the aid of the clinician's intervention, which helped assure members of the integrity of boundaries between patients, the members, although upset and agitated, demonstrated that they could manage the feelings without leaving or losing control. Dorothy at first communicated her discomfort directly, and then later metaphorically ("We have a big stomach; that is, we are stuffed with anger"). The linking of Warren and Claire served to diminish anxiety and resulted in a corrective emotional experience for Dorothy.

This example illustrates the potential volatility of patient extragroup contact. However, this group was able to convert a potential conflagration into a therapeutically positive experience. Extragroup contacts diffuse treatment boundaries and decrease a sense of safety in the treatment room. The therapeutic trade-off is one of increased opportunities to make social linkages. In contrast with groups of more psychologically sophisticated persons, members do not recognize the significance of their outside contacts except as a source of gratification or frustration, and consequently, they do not readily discuss their meetings with the hope of gaining self-understanding. Ultimately, clinicians recognize they do not control patients' meetings, and to the best of their ability, they must monitor the group interactions to minimize negative effects.

Dealing with Death

Although no precise data are available, groups with chronically ill members seem to be exposed to death more frequently than groups composed of higher functioning individuals. Deaths occur from accidents, violence (murders), suicide, and from medical illnesses. In part the deaths are a consequence of patients' problems in receiving high-quality medical care. A complex interaction occurs between access to care, providers' tendency toward dismissing medical problems in mentally ill persons, and patients' hesitation in seeking care. It is not only patients but relatives and acquaintances who die.

Sometimes it is a member who is the first to learn of another's death. The patient network is well connected, and it is not unusual for members to be knowledgeable about others, including details of their health. On occasion, particularly following a murder, the evening news informs everyone.

> *Example*: In one group, a chronically depressed widow, subsisting on Social Security Disability Insurance (SSDI), suddenly assumed the care of four early adolescent grandchildren following her daughter's murder by her estranged husband. Her daughter had been killed in front of the children. The oldest child had been pistol-whipped, and he survived only because the gun jammed.
>
> The patient's grief over her daughter's death was complicated by her responsibilities in helping the children grieve, manage their symptoms of PTSD, as well as having insufficient living space and inadequate income. She received only minimal assistance from her other adult children. More intensive case management helped solve some of the reality problems, but the patient's emotional distress remained a major focus within the group for more than a year, often stimulated as the murderer was arraigned, trial dates were set, and court appearances for the children were scheduled. Intermittent media coverage kept the event in the awareness of all members.

When a long-term member dies, the reaction within the group is quite varied. In addition to their own capacities to manage grief, members' responses reflect the cause of death and the person's linkages to the group. Relationships among members usually have not been limited to the meetings, but have spilled over into their daily lives, a phenomenon that may add poignancy to the grief.

Typical of the responses are efforts to recapture an image of the person

("Wasn't she the lady who was wearing something red the last time she came to group?") or recounting the last time contact had been made ("I had just talked with her at the hospital on Wednesday"). Some patients may turn away from death and focus on positive aspects of life, such as new births or children's accomplishments. Others will become concerned with physical ailments, and they express worries about how they are managing chronic illnesses such as diabetes or hypertension. They may wonder about the health of members who have terminated the group, or they may become philosophical ("Life is short, and you never know when you are going to go"). These responses usually contain a wish that the death might have been prevented (or at least the suffering minimized in the circumstance of someone dying with a chronic physical illness), but this does not necessarily imply a regression to archaic dependency wishes. Patients' capacities to cry can be valuable to those who may have been inhibited in exposing their tears in front of others.

Grief is not confined to the members. Therapists can be deeply affected by a member's death. The potential for countertransference responses increases under these circumstances, either in the form of not understanding metaphorical references to dying or in overinterpreting all losses as a response to the death. A clinician's capacity to contain his or her own affects in a positive fashion may enhance the overall treatment. It would be foolish to deny a sense of loss or sadness, and self-revelation may free others. A caveat is in order, however, since some charismatic therapists may artificially use these experiences to demonstrate their affective freedom, with the implication that the members are defective if they are not as emotionally open.

The Acting-Out Patient

Therapists sometimes are faced with problems stemming from patients who possess insufficient ability to contain their affects and respond with behavioral discontrol—they act out. These responses may be stimulated in the interactions during a meeting, or a patient may arrive at a session verging on the loss of control (as happens with substance abuse), which continues once inside the meeting. Problems with containment occur both within and following sessions. The term "acting out" is used here as a general descriptor of behavioral discontrol. The therapeutic task of containing behavior may take precedence over immediate understanding, but both elements require the clinician's attention.

Action is a method of communication. Freud (1914) proposed that experiences a patient has repressed and forgotten from early childhood may reappear in the form of an action, in the absence of any memory. This formulation serves as a reminder of the developmental deficits embedded in patients' actions and the insufficiency in their capacity to put memories or feelings into words. The screaming infant with a wet or soiled diaper, or a toddler having a tantrum in response to frustration, illustrates actions conveying feelings. Equivalent behaviors in adults frequently evoke negative and/or aversive responses.

When behaviors become disturbing to the therapeutic process, an effort should be made to contain the disruption. The potential for affect contagion spreading confusion throughout the group is considerable, and firm measures are needed to restore a working environment. For example, the response to tension in some groups is for members to pair off and start "side" conversations. Suddenly private discussions seem to be everywhere, and the group appears to have dissolved into fragments. In these circumstances, the therapist must move to interrupt the initial pairing discussions before disorganization takes hold.

Other behaviors also disrupt the therapeutic process. Some patients will become agitated and through their body movements create significant distractions. Members may move their chairs outside the circle, where they make noise, rattle papers, rummage through belongings, and repeatedly cough or blow their noses. At times therapists hope that the patient will tire and cease what he or she is doing (like a child will tire of throwing a tantrum), or they hope that other members will speak up to stop the behaviors. Unfortunately, the usual response is to do nothing, which leads to chaos within the group. The clinician almost always has to step in and ask the disruptive person to desist. This move is often resisted by therapists who fear that they will express their annoyance or anger too directly. Under the sway of a more nondirective ideology, there may be too great a delay. The tendency to hold off and wait should be resisted, and the therapist should take action.

Not every intervention is fully successful. A patient may become subdued for a short while and then start up again, or the therapist's efforts may fail altogether. The therapist should then consider asking the member to leave the group, either for a short period (a time-out) or for the remainder of the session.

Members will respond to this use of authority. They will communicate their responses in a multitude of channels, sometimes directly, more often in metaphor or through behavior. Not all reactions are negative, because in most instances members experience considerable relief that limits have been set. However, not uncommonly, one or more individuals who feel particularly entitled will angrily respond to what they perceive as over-control.

Members' reactions will not be limited to the particular meeting, but will carry over into following sessions. It is not a violation of confidentiality for the therapist to make reference to interactions in prior sessions in the likely event that at any particular session not everyone had been present. Because the conflict or acting out took place during the meeting, it is "public" knowledge. The therapist should make an effort to help members explore their feelings about disruptive experiences by translating metaphors into the here and now of the group. If this is done in a respectful fashion, and patients are provided sufficient space to disagree with or ignore what has been said, the therapist conveys his or her willingness to address difficult topics.

Sometimes a therapist has an uncanny experience when a patient, having missed a meeting, enters and immediately begins to discuss a family problem or cites a community event that parallels what happened in the prior session in his or her absence. In these circumstances the therapist can use the content as a segue into discussing the preceding meeting.

Acting out also happens when patients exhibit psychosis within the meeting. Patients may present with severe thought disorder and either hallucinate or discuss delusions about any aspect of the treatment situation. Not all of these behaviors are group disruptive, and members generally are tolerant of considerable expressions of psychotic or affective decompensation. However, if a person cannot be contained, or the stimulation of members' interactions seems to escalate psychotic thinking, the patient can be removed from a meeting.

A decision to remove a patient from the group seems easier under these circumstances than one in which the patient suffers from personality problems and appears to have more conscious control over behavior. Members may react with relief when an overtly ill person is asked to leave, but they are also frightened by such events because of their underlying fears that they too might become ill again. Expressions of guilt also appear as members feel responsible for stimulating the patient in a manner that led to the upsurge in his or her illness and/or removal from the meeting.

The therapist should not confine his or her attention to behavioral control, but should also be attempting to understand the underlying dynamics. A window of opportunity can exist when limits have been set and followed up with an interpretation of the basis for the disorganization. The state of the transference in the group is the most useful place to begin. A disruptive person may be the members' messenger to the therapist of his or her failure to understand or to intervene at the time of an earlier stress. A patient who enters the group in behavioral disarray may be responding to the prior session's tension.

Example: Following the departure of a therapist, a senior clinician assumed group leadership but was unsuccessful in recruiting new members. He decided to merge the group (A) into another (B) that he also led. Group B had a large roster, but a small core subgroup.

In the second merged session, seven members were present, including four members from group A. Following brief introductions because three individuals had not been present the preceding week, Ms. L (group A) irritably reported that her daughter had written her from prison requesting large quantities of clothes. This stimulated considerable excitement and several members began talking at once. The content concerned children who made demands and did not respect their parents. The therapist firmly asked that only one person speak at a time.

Momentarily the group fell silent and then the preceding theme of demanding and irresponsible children was picked up and elaborated by the four members from group A, who often talked over one another. The therapist suggested that members of group A were probably quite uneasy about joining the other group, and they had the task of meeting new people. At this point Ms. M, a group A member, asserted major leadership and acknowledged her anxiety. She then seemed to direct and contain the group while they all discussed problems of change and loss. The meeting ended with a comment that it was good to have so many people present to listen.

In this meeting, the anxiety stirred by melding the two groups was stimulated by the theme of resentment over demanding children. The initial disruption was firmly checked, but the intervention was only temporarily effective, and the salient theme continued. When the therapist focused on the anxiety (without interpreting the metaphor), members were able to examine experiences of loss (their own groups) and anxiety over change and sharing, which they then were able to utilize in a more conscious and direct fashion. The session ended on a positive note.

Not all stresses are successfully managed during a meeting, and consequently patients "act" outside the boundaries of the meeting. Phone calls and visits to the clinic or to the emergency room are common enactments of increased anxiety. Many patients do not consciously make connections between what has happened in their treatment and their behavioral disturbance, and they may not inform other professionals of their membership in a group. As a consequence, treatment decisions are made without appropriate collaboration. On other occasions, patients may be quite aware of withholding information about the group or present the treatment as antitherapeutic, as a way of retaliation or of finding a "good parent." Some splitting is inevitable, and clinicians will do well to avoid being ensnared by patients' defensive operations.

Acting out may lead to serious consequences for the patient. Failure to contain anxieties in one setting can lead to acting out in another. Groups simulate aspects of an individual's family, and it is not surprising, therefore, that a person's family might become the target for group-induced frustrations.

> *Example*: Henry, a man diagnosed in DSM-IV Cluster B of action-oriented personality disorders, became upset with a woman cotherapist, whom he perceived as not paying him sufficient attention. Following the session, he became involved in a violent argument with his estranged wife's boyfriend, which ended in a physical fight. As a result, Henry was arrested and sent to jail for 30 days.

The group therapists explored their countertransference responses to Henry, which included anger, guilt, and shame. He had been a difficult member, and they had often wished that he might terminate. Although not knowingly acting on those feelings, the clinicians felt a degree of remorse as well as pleasure at Henry's punishment. Supervision was particularly useful in assisting the therapists to address these complex feelings.

> *Example*: Thor, a foreign-born man diagnosed with schizophrenia, attended regularly but spoke infrequently and then usually in response to being directly addressed. He often was difficult to understand, because his language difficulty was compounded by his psychotic thought disorder.
> Thor missed several sessions and then was brought to a meeting by one of the clinic support staff. He had obviously lost weight and appeared confused. When asked what had been happening, Thor seemed unable to provide a clear explanation. He abruptly left the session. The therapist considered following Thor, but desisted. Shortly thereafter, Thor exhibited himself in the city square and was arrested. He was remanded to the prison psychiatric facility. The therapist experienced guilt at not having appreciated the urgency of Thor's illness and failing to respond to the obvious signs of deterioration in his clinical state.

Although the emphasis has been on exploring the dynamic basis for acting out, therapists also should consider the value of pharmacological intervention. In retrospect, clearly Thor was disorganized, and steps to medicate him and/or arrange hospitalization would have been a propitious action.

One of the clinician's functions is to serve as a container. By being alert to a regression and suggesting that medication might be useful—the actual prescription can be arranged following the session unless there is an emergency—the therapist indicates a sense of responsibility and containment. This may have a calming effect throughout the entire group.

Members' subsequent associations to other experiences in which calming or soothing interactions occurred can serve to confirm such hypotheses.

Another serious problem is that of patients bringing weapons to the group. Fortunately this occurs infrequently, but if a therapist knows that a patient has either a knife or a gun on his or her person in the meeting, that information should be treated as an emergency. The sense of safety in the group is altered and must be addressed. In many instances patients carry weapons as self-protection and have little intention of using it in an aggressive manner. For example, when a change in clinical condition (e.g., an emergence of paranoia and fears of being attacked) is the basis for carrying a knife or gun, the potential for misinterpretation of in-group transactions exists, with a possibly lethal outcome.

In these circumstances the patient can be invited to give the weapon to the therapist, or take it to a designated place outside of the treatment room. The therapist should make simple explanation that weapons are not permitted in the treatment setting. If a patient is too frightened to part with the weapon, he or she should be asked to leave the group. This step should be taken even if information emerges that the patient has been carrying the weapon for a long period. The fact that the information is no longer secret suggests a change in clinical status that requires exploration.

Therapists are often as affected as members in these clinical situations. The potential for countertransference responses is increased in unfamiliar or threatening situations. Therapists may find themselves distracted, immersed in their own reverie or anger. These emotional responses may be used to gain a greater understanding of the clinical situation, for clinicians can explore their own responses to determine if the affect is primarily a product of their own personality and past life experiences or if it would be an expected response to the behavior.

Recommendations in this section have focused on certain conditions in which therapists might need to assert their authority and act without the benefit of much time to fully evaluate a situation. Even if the action is assessed within the treatment framework, therapists might experience discomfort and become uncertain of their therapeutic judgment. If regular supervision is not available, consultation with a trusted colleague can serve to disentangle the various strands and help therapists regain their balance.

SUMMARY

This chapter has examined aspects of the group that emerge in the treatment process of groups for the chronically mentally ill. Patients' discussion of medication carries several levels of meaning, including metaphorical messages about either an individual or the entire group.

When dreams are presented, the clinicians assesses the patients' capacities to work with various levels of meaning. Dreams will reveal a good deal about patients' perceptions of themselves within the context of the group. This may be useful information to the clinician, even when he or she decides not to intervene.

The model of a flexibly bound group normalizes the presence of peripheral members. Nevertheless, there are important emotional responses on the part of individuals who comprise the core group and those in the peripheral subgroup that require attention. Achieving a balance that respects the feelings of both subgroups is an important element in the continuing life of the group.

A multitude of difficult clinical situations arise from working with patients in a group setting. The monopolizing masochist can alienate others and evoke countertransferences that may be burdensome. Complications of extragroup contacts are discussed in the context of subgrouping and silence. At times, limits may be necessary to protect the group.

Responses to deaths of group members, their families, or their acquaintances are woven into the fabric of the group. Deaths due to illness, suicide, or homicide are frequently discussed and are more prevalent in the chronically ill population.

Acting out is a communication about the interaction and patients' difficulty in verbally expressing themselves. It is to be expected as an important element in the continuing therapeutic process. Management depends on the capacities of the members and the level of group development. Therapists are often hard pressed to find useful interventions, but the integrity of the group should be the paramount consideration unless there is substantial danger to the individual(s).

FOURTEEN

CONCLUSION

*We still believe that it is not only helpful but
indispensable for psychotherapeutic success to study the
patient's and psychiatrist's mutual relationships in terms
of their repetitional characteristics. But we keenly feel
that this should not be done to the point of neglecting to
scrutinize the reality of the actual experience between
therapist and patient in its own right.*

—FROMM-REICHMANN (1950, p. 4)

This is a book about the clinical care of chronically ill patients in groups. I have attempted to provide clinicians with sufficient theoretical and practical information that they can begin to think about their work with groups of these individuals from a new perspective. This book represents a beginning. There is no substitute for clinical work and appropriate supervision. Indeed, as I have noted in Chapter 6, in order for a group program to survive, therapists must receive the same respect and care from colleagues and administrators as they provide for patients.

Treatment outcome has not been addressed. Research in the field is rudimentary (Chapter 3), and a multitude of factors confound design and implementation of research. Naturalistic studies have focused on the long-term outcomes for schizophrenic patients, but they represent only a portion of the chronically ill population. Studies of patients discharged from state hospitals have become dated, because patients no longer reside in institutions for extended periods and may only temporarily receive treatment in hospitals before they are rapidly discharged into the community. Patients' impairments and the availability and variability of services and levels of care in the community are considerable. These elements interrelate, and their complexity assures us that research will not make quantum leaps to provide global answers.

Delivery of mental health services is undergoing major change, and the view of the future is clouded by many social and political imponderables. Many patients will require treatment throughout their lives. Some can be sustained with brief medication visits and social relationships that enable them to lead reasonably satisfactory lives. Others can benefit from peer-led support groups. Still others, who are the subject of this book, have significant social deficits that can be modified by participation in extended periods of group psychotherapy. The treatment intensity need not be great, but care will require the availability of continuing social networks that enhance patients' quality of life and prevent relapse.

The model described here is flexible. Patients can belong to a group for several decades, which may sustain and even strengthen their social skills and capacities to develop satisfying interpersonal relationships. Julian Leff, who works with schizophrenic patients and their families using a psychoeducational model, commented in a personal communication (1992) that patients and their families seem unable to sustain the learning they have achieved if treatment is terminated. Therefore, he arranges for his patients to be seen at intervals for many years. Similarly, group patients benefit from not terminating but continuing in their treatment.

THE THERAPIST'S EXPERIENCE

The many barriers to clinicians sustaining their work with this population have been discussed earlier in this volume. Even in optimal settings, not all therapists find themselves suited to a leadership role. Those who do find themselves undergoing a transformation in their appreciation of the "lived-in world" of their patients. One therapist observed that when she began coleading a group, she was anxious and ill prepared to become truly acquainted with the patients. Nevertheless, she learned that they suffered stresses and conflicts similar to her own. She now experiences them as persons, like herself, who are trying to make the best of their lives.

For several years medical students were offered a 6-week elective in observing a group of chronically ill patients. The students served as operators of a video camera and, following the session, met with the therapist for a detailed review of the tape. These were mainly interested and motivated students who, even in this relatively brief period came to "know" the group members in a way that may have stimulated their interest in working with this patient population in the future. One talented but naive student acted on her feelings of involvement and baked cookies, which she brought for the patients at her final meeting. She too had become linked to the members, seeing them not as symptoms but as people suffering under the burden of their illness.

Unfortunately, there are only limited numbers of well-trained clinicians who gain such self-understanding that would lead to compassionate and continued interest in working with chronically mentally ill persons. The rewards can be considerable in observing patients manage difficult situations with greater dignity. A clinician looks back and begins to appreciate the small changes that have taken place over extended periods. There is less turmoil in patients' lives, and conflict don't seem as pressured. Some of these changes will be described in the patients' own words in the following section.

Therapists often are startled by the intensity of their emotional responses when they discontinue working with a group. On occasion, trainees choose to remain with a group beyond the necessary training requirements in response to recognition of both their attachment and therapeutic value to the group, as well as their positive learning experience. For many trainees, who initially were asked to conduct groups as part of a educational requirement, the terminations stir sadness and surprise at the feelings of loss that they experience. These feelings are intensified manyfold for staff members who depart after working with a group for a number of years. Those terminations are often accompanied by considerable grief.

Patients develop strong attachments to their therapists. They send their therapists Christmas cards, which reflects an expenditure of precious financial resources. Trainees comment on this phenomenon, noting that there are a disproportionate number of cards from group patients in comparison with similar individuals they treat in a dyadic format. In one of my groups, the patients surprised me with a gift of a bottle of liquor at Christmastime. All six members, who were supported by public funds, had contributed to purchase the gift! In addition, the members had chosen the most vulnerable and sensitive member to purchase the accompanying card, which reflected the others' sensitivity to this patient's need to be seen as responsible. This level of comradery and collaboration among the members was not as clearly apparent in their group interactions. The bottle of liquor was left in plain view in my home workspace for several months before I consciously became aware of the continuing pleasure I received from that gift.

PATIENTS' VIEWS

I will conclude this book with reports of patients' experiences of their group membership. Group members were asked to write a report of their experience in treatment, commenting on the aspects that they liked and felt were useful, and those that they disliked or found not to be beneficial. The written responses were sparse, and as a result, therapists were asked to interview their patients, asking the same questions and, when necessary, asking for elaboration. More than 30 individuals provided written responses or participated in interviews.

The responses enumerating positive elements in belonging to a group reflected a surprising range in patients' capacities to "explain" their treatment experience. Almost all of the patients commented on the value of listening to others' stories and feeling that they were not alone with their illness. They often mentioned the positive impact on themselves of telling their stories and having others listen. These responses were poignant confirmations of the group therapeutic factors of catharsis and universality found in more formal research (Butler & Fuhrimann, 1980; Yalom, 1985; Bloch & Crouch, 1985).

Some individuals were able to describe their experiences in considerable psychological depth. One patient, diagnosed with schizoaffective disorder and having made substantial progress, described her perceptions of how the group had evolved. She said that initially, just listening to others' stories and telling her own had been very useful, but the group had taken a different turn more recently, and members began to look at their own relationships. She said that this was hard, but it was very helpful. A small number of individuals went beyond relationship factors and provided comments about their treatment goals, which included insight into behaviors that they wished to change. Their comments were framed in terms of learning to listen and respect others and to contain angry feelings that caused them interpersonal difficulties. They could be understood as developing insight.

The following are representative samples of patients' responses obtained either from their written responses or their therapists' verbatim notes. The errors in spelling and grammar are not edited in order to convey the patients' presentation of their experience.

> "It is helpful to listen to others problems and this calms me and helps me understand how I feel. I like meeting with the ladies and feel others care."

> "Everyone seem like they understand every thing I have been through with and I feel free to talk with them. . . . Being with people who understand what one goes through whose nerves aren't like they're suppose to be. To express my fears, anxieties without someone laughing at me or saying it's all in my head. It helps me to deal with the atrocities that have besieged me by evil people since 1983."

> "I believe in coming to group, because it give me something to do. It occupies my time."

"I like coming to therapy groups because it gives me a chance to talk to other people and talk through my problems as unimportant as they might seem to me and others. It lets me see that I [am] not alone in the world."

"They listen and give you feedback and what you say in group stays in group."

"Several things were helpful. I'm not the only one with worries and cares that have been in my life that other people have. I used to think that I was alone in my worries. I didn't think there were people in my age that were going through similar things that I had. I believe going to group and talking about certain things and listening to others talk helps me."

Some patients' responses reflected their relationship with the therapist, and the members seemed secondary or absent.

"The first day I went to group, I was nervous when I met Dr. [X], I didn't know what he would be like. I have got over being nervous after I got to know him real well. It has help me a lot being in group therapy. Dr. [X] has helped me a lot."

"I thank Dr. [X] for the time and courage that he listen to us as we discuss our problem to one another and me in group session."

One woman, diagnosed with borderline personality disorder and attending the group for 12 years, commented only about the therapist. She responded to the therapist's request, "Please describe the most helpful thing to you as a group member" with "You!" The interviewer's efforts to ask about the members was responded to with more about the therapist:

"I trust you. I can talk to you. It's OK [coming to the group], I see faces that I know and you are here. If I see your face, I'm OK."

This patient, however, often interacted with the others in a friendly and helpful fashion.

After describing how it was helpful to know that he was not alone with his problems, a schizophrenic man who had been a group member for 14 years, said,

"My attitude has changed a whole lot for the better. I have more feelings toward people. It all stems from conversations that come out in the group and I worry about some of the people in the group like [patient]. Before I couldn't care. If you say something out of the way to me I would give it back to you in full force. My appearance has changed. Before I wouldn't care. I was wild. I was alcoholic. Me and [patient] talked about alcohol and how it was, and I talked to you about it. I don't drink anymore."

Criticisms of the therapy were sparse, which may have reflected patients' unwillingness to be critical of the treatment directly to their caregiver. The following represent the patients' responses:

> "Talking over your head. I don't know anything about the different medicines."
> "Not always feeling a part of group."
> "This cussing a lot."
> "Need help expressing my feelings."
> "Sometimes people talk about things that aren't material to me—like grandbabies."
> "I thought [patient] was getting snotty toward you. I got real mad at him. He got hateful to you. To get that mad wasn't helpful. I didn't like that."

The more limited responses suggesting ways that group treatment could be more helpful were limited to two individuals: One person wished the therapists would speak more often, and the other suggested that the group meet twice weekly.

The responses may reflect group members' lack of sophistication, but they are capable of conveying their experience in plain and understandable language. The treatment appears to reflect members' emphasis on diminishing their pervasive sense of being different and alone. The interaction of the group structure with the therapist's skills and the patients' extensive and often global disabilities provides for meaningful opportunities for patients to feel less isolated and more connected to a social network.

The following is the most articulate report, provided by a 46-year-old single man diagnosed with schizoaffective disorder. He had a series of hospitalizations beginning at age 38, but he had not been hospitalized for over a year, when he began group treatment three years previously. The patient wrote,

> "I entered group on a wave of expectation about one year after my last hospitalization. There have been seven in all. For a while it seemed like a call. I'm doing much better since the last, hopefully it's over and a thing of the past.
> "Group therefor appears to be an effective tool in my overall therapy which also includes individual psychotherapy. Though I whine and complain and threaten to leave, it has helped me be more assertive and confident of myself. Growth is so slow however, and I

am so impatient that I often feel nothing is happening. It's difficult to be patient because there are so many things I would like to be doing. I see people who enjoy life and glory in being alive. This often makes my heartache because I can't join in. I turn to alcohol or drugs and enter a subterranean existence which is better than no existence at all. The only other alternative for me is working myself in therapy and on my own. This has been the most difficult undertaking I can conceive of and I could have done better. There is always room for improvement but I have no other choice.

"The other members of our group are mixed bags of pluses and minuses in their own right. There are four other members and I am in a love/hate relationship with each one. Over the past one and one half years I've gotten to know them pretty well and I love each one. They say that the true test of love for a person is if you would ultimately die for them. As for my friends in group I don't think would go that far, but I would cut off a finger if that would bring them to health. As for at times hating them this is due to my myopic perspective. Bad nerves, low attitude and my own prejudices. It's not that they are bad but frustrating and difficult for me to deal with.

"I often think I am nearly there. I think that until the next depression comes around anyway. Then I can't see the forest for the trees. I have a little talent in a number of areas. I'm just too hateful."

SUMMARY

Perhaps this book is about xenophobia. Chronically mentally ill patients are "different." They often communicate in ways that are difficult to understand. They have difficulty expressing their feelings. When asked directly to talk about their experiences, their capacities to do so vary widely. Moreover, at times they express feelings and impulses that may seem alien or unfathomable to their caregivers. It is not surprising that the mentally ill are stigmatized.

It is my hope that the therapist working in the group setting will begin to make sense and gain an appreciation of the members' inner experience. Clinicians learn about patients' struggles to survive and to enjoy their lives to whatever extent they can, taking into account the biological, interpersonal, and social elements they face. In the process, they learn that they are not fundamentally different from their patients. And so the gulf between patients and therapists closes.

NOTES

CHAPTER 2

1. Arizona, Colorado, Hawaii, Maryland, New Jersey, New York, North Carolina, Ohio, Pennsylvania, and Texas were the 10 states examined in the study.

CHAPTER 3

1. A recent survey revealed that only a very few therapists include schizophrenic or bipolar patients in their ordinary outpatient treatment groups. It was estimated that less than 1% of the patients in the groups were diagnosed with schizophrenia and were receiving medication. Only about 2% of the group members were diagnosed with mania (Stone et al., 1991).

2. The six studies reviewed by these authors are cited in the references: Shattan et al.(1966), Levene et al. (1970), Purvis and Miskimins (1970), O'Brien et al.(1972), Herz et al.(1974), and Claghorn et al.(1974).

CHAPTER 4

1. Only 4% of the study group were employed.

2. Assessment of social networks and role functioning of chronically mentally ill individuals has been difficult. Objective and subjective measures are used to evaluate the quantitative and qualitative aspects of kin and nonkin relationships. Among objective measures are strategies that count the size, type, and accessibility of contacts a patient might have in a specified period. The type of contact would include the number of different activities with network members. Other studies include measures of the frequency of emotional or practical support provided by network members to the patient, or, conversely, the supports provided by the patient to others. Subjective assessments might include bimodal ratings (e.g., very pleased or displeased) for any of these relationships. Inquiries into the person's wishes for different types of relationships or the researcher's evaluation of the response to interview situations or to life stressors can be part of the database.

3. High expressed emotion appears to be a rather stable characteristic, and in two reports, 75% or more of the families remained high on a repeat evaluation (Leff et al., 1982, Hogarty et al., 1986).

4. In a study of 35 diabetic subjects, glucose control was significantly predicted by the critical-comments component of expressed emotion, suggesting that this construct is not specific to psychiatric patients (Koenigsberg et al., 1993).

CHAPTER 5

1. A spindown is a cost-containment measure in which patients pay monthly a predetermined amount of money on medical–pharmacy services before they are eligible to be supported by public funds.

CHAPTER 6

1. Commercial videotapes are available to demonstrate aspects of group treatment. More detailed information can be obtained through the American Group Psychotherapy Association, 25 East 21st Street, New York, NY 10010.

REFERENCES

Adelman, S. A. (1985). Pills as transitional objects: A dynamic understanding of the use of medication in psychotherapy. *Psychiatry, 48,* 246–253.

Agazarian, Y., & Janoff, S. (1993). Systems theory and small groups. In H. I. Kaplan & B. J. Sadock (Eds.), *Comprehensive Group Psychotherapy* (3rd ed., pp. 32–44). Baltimore: Williams & Wilkins.

Alexander, F. (1946). Individual psychotherapy. *Psychosomatic Medicine, 8,* 110–115.

Amador, X. F., Flaum, M., Andreasen, N. C., Strauss, D. H., Yale, S. A., Clark, S. C., & Gorman, J. M. (1994). Awareness of illness in schizophrenia and schizoaffective and mood disorders. *Archives of General Psychiatry, 51,* 826–836.

Amador, X. F., Strauss, D. H., Yale, S. A., Flaum, M. M., Endicott, J., & Gorman, J. M. (1993). Assessment of insight in psychosis. *American Journal of Psychiatry, 150,* 873–879.

American Psychiatric Association. (1980). *Diagnostic and Statistical Manual of Mental Disorders* (3rd ed.). Washington, DC: Author.

American Psychiatric Association. (1994). *Diagnostic and Statistical Manual of Mental Disorders* (4th ed.). Washington, DC: Author.

Ananth, J., Vandewater, S., Kamal, M., Brodsky, A., Gamal, R., & Miller, M. (1989). Missed diagnosis of substance abuse in psychiatric patients. *Hospital and Community Psychiatry, 40,* 297–299.

Anthony, W. A., & Jansen, M. A. (1984). Predicting the vocational capacity of the chronically mentally ill: Research and policy implications. *American Psychologist, 39,* 537–544.

Aronson, M. L. (1975). The leader's role in focusing. In Z. A. Liff (Ed.), *The Leader in the Group* (pp. 151–160). New York: Jason Aronson.

Aronson, T. A., Shukla, S., Gujavarty, K., Hoff, A., DiBuno, M., & Khan, E. (1988). Relapse in delusional depression: A retrospective study of the course of treatment. *Comprehensive Psychiatry, 29,* 12–21.

Ashback, C., & Schermer, V. L. (1987). *Object Relations, the Self and the Group.* London: Routledge & Kegan Paul.

Astrachan, B. M., Flynn, H. R., Geller, J. D., & Harvey, H. H. (1970). Systems approach to day hospitalization. *Archives of General Psychiatry, 22,* 550–559.

Bachrach, L. L. (1986). Dimension of disability in the chronic mentally ill. *Hospital and Community Psychiatry, 37,* 981–982.

Bachrach, L. L. (1988). Defining chronic mental illness: A concept paper. *Hospital and Community Psychiatry, 39,* 383–388.

Bachrach, L. L. (1992). What we know about homelessness among mentally ill persons: An analytical review and commentary. *Hospital and Community Psychiatry, 42,* 453–464.

Bachrach, L. L., & Lamb, H. R. (1989). What have we learned from deinstitutionalization? *Psychiatric Annals, 19,* 12–21.

Baldessarini, R. J. (1989). Current status of antidepressants: Clinical pharmacology and therapy. *Journal of Clinical Psychiatry, 50,* 117–126.

Barnes, R. F., Mason, J. C., Greer, C., & Ray, F. T. (1983). Medical illness in chronic psychiatric outpatients. *General Hospital Psychiatry, 5,* 191–195.

Battegay, R., & von Marschall, R. (1978). Results of long-term group psychotherapy with schizophrenics. *Comprehensive Psychiatry, 19,* 349–353.

Beck, J. C. (1969). Outpatient group therapy of the poor. In J. H. Masserman (Ed.), *Current Psychiatric Therapies: 1969* (pp. 241–244). New York: Grune & Stratton.

Bellack, A. S. (1992). Cognitive rehabilitation for schizophrenia: Is it possible? Is it necessary? *Schizophrenia Bulletin, 18,* 43–50.

Bellack, A. S., Morrison, R. L., & Mueser, K. T. (1989). Social problem solving in schizophrenia. *Schizophrenia Bulletin, 15,* 101–116.

Bennis, W. G., & Shepard, H. A. (1956). A theory of group development. *Human Relations, 9,* 415–437.

Bergman, H. C., & Harris, M. (1985). Substance abuse among young adult chronic patients. *Psychosocial Rehabilitation Journal, 9,* 49–54.

Bion, W. R. (1961). *Experiences in Groups.* New York: Basic Books.

Black, D. W. (1988). Mortality in schizophrenia. The Iowa record-linkage study: A comparison with general population mortality. *Psychosomatics, 29,* 55–60.

Blau, D., & Zilbach, J. J. (1954). The use of group psychotherapy in posthospitalization treatment. *American Journal of Psychiatry, 111,* 244–248.

Blaustein, M. (1985). Introduction and overview: Residential care and treatment of the chronic mental patient. *Psychiatric Annals, 15,* 633–638.

Bleuler, E. (1911). *Dementia Praecox or the Group of Schizophrenias* (J. Zinkin, Trans.). New York: International Universities Press, 1950.

Bloch, S., & Crouch E. (1985). *Therapeutic Factors in Group Psychotherapy.* Oxford: Oxford University Press.

Bouhuys, A. L., & Van den Hoofdakker, R. H. (1993). A longitudinal study of interaction of a psychiatrist and severely depressed patients based on observed behavior: An ethological approach of interpersonal theories of depressions. *Journal of Affective Disorders, 27,* 87–99.

Brady, J. P. (1984). Social skills training for psychiatric patients, I: Concepts, methods and clinical results. *American Journal of Psychiatry, 141,* 333–340.

Braff, D. L., & Geyer, M. A. (1990). Sensorimotor gating and schizophrenia: Human and animal model studies. *Archives of General Psychiatry, 47,* 181–188.

Breakey, W. R., Fischer, P. J., Kramer, M., Nestadt, G., Romanoski, A. J., Ross, A., Royall, R. M., & Stine, O. C. (1989). Health and mental health problems of homeless men and women in Baltimore. *Journal of the American Medical Association, 262,* 1352–1357.

Breier, A., Schreiber, J. L., Dyer, J., & Pickar, D. (1991). National Institute of Mental Health longitudinal study of chronic schizophrenia. *Archives of General Psychiatry, 48,* 239–248.

Breier, A., & Strauss, J. S. (1984). The role of social relationships in the recovery from psychotic disorders. *American Journal of Psychiatry, 141,* 949–955.

Brown, G. W., Carstairs, G. M., & Topping, G. (1958). Post hospital adjustment of chronic mental patients. *Lancet, 2,* 685–689.

Brown, G. W., Monck, E. M., Carstairs, G. M., Wing, J. K. (1962). Influence of family life on the course of schizophrenic illness. *British Journal of Preventative and Social Medicine, 16,* 55–68.

Brown, P. L. (1988, July 16). Troubled millions heed call of self-help groups. *New York Times,* p. A1.

Buckley, P. (1986). Supportive psychotherapy: A neglected treatment. *Psychiatric Annals, 16,* 515–521.

Butler, T., & Fuhriman, A. (1980). Patient perspective on the curative process: A comparison of day treatment and outpatient psychotherapy groups. *Small Group Behavior, 11,* 371–388.

Cancro, R. (1983). Individual psychotherapy in the treatment of chronic schizophrenic patients. *American Journal of Psychotherapy, 37,* 493–501.

Carone, B. J., Harrow, M., & Westermeyer, J. F. (1991). Posthospital course and outcome in schizophrenia. *Archives of General Psychiatry, 48,* 247–253.

Caton, C. L. M., Gralnick, A., Bender, S., & Simon, R. (1989). Young chronic patients and substance abuse. *Hospital and Community Psychiatry, 40,* 1037–1040.

Cerbone, M. J. A., Mayo, J. A., Cuthbertson, M. A., & O'Connell, R. A. (1992). Group therapy as an adjunct to medication in the management of bipolar affective disorder. *Group, 16,* 174–187.

Chen, A. (1991). Noncompliance in community psychiatry: A review of clinical interventions. *Hospital and Community Psychiatry, 42,* 282–287.

Chess, S., & Hassibi, M. (1986). *Principles and Practice of Child Psychiatry* (2nd ed.). New York: Plenum Press.

Christmas, J. J. (1966). Group therapy with the disadvantaged. In J. H. Masserman (Ed.), *Current Psychiatric Therapies* (pp. 163–171). New York: Grune & Stratton.

Claghorn, J. L., Johnstone, E. E., Cook, T. H., & Itschner, L. (1974). Group therapy and maintenance treatment of schizophrenics. *Archives of General Psychiatry, 31,* 361–365.

Cooper, E. J. (1978). The pre-group: The narcissistic phase of group development with the severely disturbed patient. In L. R. Wolberg & M. L. Aronson (Eds.), *Group Therapy 1978* (pp. 60–71). New York: Stratton Intercontinental Medical Book.

Coryell, W., Keller, M., Lavori, P., & Endicott, J. (1990). Affective syndromes, psychotic features and prognosis: I. Depression. *Archives of General Psychiatry, 47,* 651–657.

Coryell, W., Scheftner, Keller, M., Endicott, J., Maser, J., & Klerman, G.I. (1993). The enduring psychosocial consequences of mania and depression. *American Journal of Psychiatry, 150,* 720–727.

Coryell, W., & Tsuang, M. T. (1982). Primary unipolar depression and the prognostic importance of delusions. *Archives of General Psychiatry, 39,* 1181–1184.

Davies, M. A., Bromet, E. J., Schulz, S. C., Dunn, L. O., & Morgenstern, M. (1989). Community adjustment of chronic schizophrenic patients in urban and rural settings. *Hospital and Community Psychiatry, 40,* 824–830.

Davies, M. J. (1967). Nightmares and psychopathology. In H. Kellerman (Ed.), *The Nightmare: Psychological and Biological Foundations* (pp. 217–228). New York: Columbia University Press.

de Bosset, F. (1982). Core group: A psychotherapeutic model in an outpatient clinic. *Canadian Journal of Psychiatry, 27,* 123–126.

de Bosset, F. (1988). A comparison of homogeneous and heterogeneous group psychotherapy models for chronic psychiatric outpatients. *Psychiatry Journal University of Ottawa, 13,* 212–214.

de Bosset, F. (1991). Group psychotherapy in chronic psychiatric outpatients. *International Journal of Group Psychotherapy, 41,* 65–78.

Dement, W. (1955). Dream recall and eye movements during sleep in schizophrenics and normals. *Journal of Nervous and Mental Disease, 122,* 263–269.

Dixon, N. F. (1979). *On the Psychology of Military Incompetence.* London: Futura Publications.

Donlon, P. T., Rada, R. T., & Knight, S. W. (1973). A therapeutic aftercare setting for "refractory" chronic schizophrenic patients. *American Journal of Psychiatry, 130,* 682–684.

Drake, R. E., & Wallach, M. A. (1989). Substance abuse among the chronic mentally ill. *Hospital and Community Psychiatry, 40,* 1041–1046.

Dubovsky, S. L., & Thomas, M. (1992). Psychotic depression: Advances in conceptualization and treatment. *Hospital and Community Psychiatry, 43,* 1189–1198.

Durkin, H. E. (1957). Toward a common basis for group dynamics: Group and therapeutic processes in group psychotherapy. *International Journal of Group Psychotherapy, 7,* 115–130.

Durkin, H. E. (1964). *The Group in Depth.* New York: International Universities Press.

Emerick, R. E. (1989). Group demographics in the mental patient movement: Group location, age, and size as structural factors. *Community Mental Health Journal, 25,* 277–300.

Englander, T. R. (1989). *The Facilitating Environment, Cohesion, and the Con-*

tract in Group Psychotherapy. Unpublished doctoral thesis, The Fielding Institute, Santa Barbara, CA.

Erickson, D. H., Beiser, M., Iacono, W. G., Fleming, J. A. E., & Lin, T. (1989). The role of social relationships in the course of first-episode schizophrenia and affective psychosis. *American Journal of Psychiatry, 146,* 1456–1461.

Erikson, E. H. (1963). *Childhood and Society* (2nd ed.). New York: Norton.

Ezriel, H. (1973). Psychoanalytic group therapy. In L. R. Wolberg & E. K. Schwartz (Eds.), *Group Therapy 1973: An Overview* (pp. 183–210). New York: Stratton Intercontinental Medical Book.

Falloon, I. R. H., Boyd, J. L., McGill, C. W., Razoni, J., Moss, H. B., & Gilderman, H. A. (1982). Family management in the prevention of exacerbations of schizophrenia. *New England Journal of Medicine, 306,* 1437–1444.

Feinberg, L., Koresko, R. L., Gottlieb, F., & Wender, P. H. (1964). Sleep electroencephalographic and eye-movement patterns in schizophrenic patients. *Comprehensive Psychiatry, 5,* 44–53.

Feldberg, T. M. (1958). Treatment of "borderline" psychotics in groups of neurotic patients. *International Journal of Group Psychotherapy, 8,* 76–84.

Frank, E., Kupfer, D. J., Perel, J. M., Cornes, C., Jarrett, D. B., Mallinger, A. G., Thase, M. E., McEachran, A. B., & Grochocinski, V. I. (1990). Three-year outcomes for maintenance therapies in recurrent depression. *Archives of General Psychiatry, 47,* 1093–1099.

Freud, S. (1905). Fragment of an analysis of a case of hysteria. In J. Strachey (Ed. & Trans.), *The Standard Edition of the Complete Psychological Works of Sigmund Freud* (Vol. 7, pp. 1–122). London: Hogarth Press, 1957.

Freud, S. (1910). The future propsects of psychoanalytic theory. In J. Strachey (Ed. &Trans.), *The Standard Edition of the Complete Psychological Works of Sigmund Freud* (Vol. 11, pp. 139–151). London: Hogarth Press, 1957.

Freud, S. (1914). Remembering, repeating and working-through: Further recommendations of the technique of psycho-analysis. In J. Strachey (Ed. & Trans.), *The Standard Edition of the Complete Psychological Works of Sigmund Freud* (Vol. 12, pp. 145–156). London: Hogarth Press, 1958.

Freud, S. (1915). Observations on transference love. In J. Strachey (Ed. & Trans.), *The Standard Edition of the Complete Psychological Works of Sigmund Freud* (Vol. 12, pp. 157–170). London: Hogarth Press, 1958).

Freud, S. (1921). Group psychology and the analysis of the ego. In J. Strachey (Ed. & Trans.), *The Standard Edition of the Complete Psychologial Works of Sigmund Freud* (Vol. 18, pp. 69–143). London: Hogarth Press, 1955.

Friedman, L. (1988). *The Anatomy of Psychotherapy.* Hillsdale, NJ: Analytic Press.

Fromm-Reichmann, F. (1950). *Principles of Intensive Psychotherapy.* Chicago: University of Chicago Press.

Fyer, A. J., & Sandberg, D. (1988). Pharmacologic treatment of panic disorder and agoraphobia. In A. J. Frances & R. E. Hales (Eds.), *Review of Psychiatry* (Vol. 7, pp. 88–120). Washington: American Psychiatric Press.

Galenter, M. (1988). Zealous self-help groups as adjuncts to psychiatric treatment: A study of Recovery, Inc. *American Journal of Psychiatry, 145,* 1248–1253.

Galenter, M. (1990). Cults and zealous self-help movements: A psychiatric perspective. *American Journal of Psychiatry, 147,* 543–551.

Gifford, S., & MacKenzie, J. (1948). A review of literature on group treatment of psychoses. *Disease of the Nervous System, 9,* 19–24.

Gilligan, C. (1982). *In a Different Voice: Psychological Theory and Women's Development.* Cambridge MA: Harvard University Press.

Glatzer, H. T. (1965). Aspects of transference in group psychotherapy. *International Journal of Group Psychotherapy, 15,* 167–176.

Goering, P. N., Lancee, W. J., & Freeman, S. J. J. (1992). Marital support and recovery from depression. *British Journal of Psychiatry, 160,* 76–82.

Goldberg, R. S., Riba, M., & Tasman, A. (1991). Psychiatrists' attitudes toward prescribing medication for patients treated by nonmedical psychotherapists. *Hospital and Community Psychiatry, 42,* 276–280.

Goldman, H. H., Gattozzi, A. A., & Taube, C. (1981). Defining and counting the chronically mentally ill. *Hospital and Community Psychiatry, 32,* 21–27.

Goldstein, M. J. (1990). Psychosocial factors relating to etiology and course of schizophrenia. In M. J. Herz, S. J. Keith, & J. P. Docherty (Eds.), *Handbook of Schizophrenia: Psychosocial Treatment of Schizophrenia* (Vol. 4, pp. 1–23). New York: Elsevier.

Goldstrom, I., & Manderscheid, R. (1972). The chronically mentally ill: A descriptive analysis from the Uniform Client Data Instrument. *Community Support Services Journal, 2,* 4–9.

Gorman, J. M., & Papp, L. A. (1990). Chronic anxiety: Deciding the length of treatment. *Journal of Clinical Psychiatry, 51*(Suppl. 1), 11–15.

Greenberg J. R., & Mitchell, S. A. (1983). *Object Relations in Psychoanalytic Theory.* Cambridge, MA: Harvard University Press.

Greenspan, S. I., & Pollock G. H. (Eds.). (1980). *The Course of Life. Psychoanalytic Contributions Toward Understanding Personality Development: Vol. III. Adulthood and the Aging Process.* Washington, DC: U.S. Department of Health and Human Services.

Grob, G. N. (1994). *The Mad Among Us: A History of Care of America's Mentally Ill.* New York: Free Press.

Grossman, L. S., Harrow, M., Goldberg, J. F., & Fichtner, C. G. (1991). Outcome of schizoaffective disorder at two long-term follow-ups: Comparisons with outcome of schizophrenia and affective disorders. *American Journal of Psychiatry, 148,* 1359–1365.

Gruenberg, E. M. (1967). The social breakdown syndrome—some origins. *American Journal of Psychiatry, 123,* 1481–1489.

Grunebaum, H., & Solomon L. (1987). Peer relationships, self-esteem and the self. *International Journal of Group Psychotherapy, 37,* 475–513.

Guze, S. B., & Robins, E. (1970). Suicide and primary affective disorders. *British Journal of Psychiatry, 117,* 437–438.

Harding, C. M., Brooks, G. W., Ashikaga, T., Strauss, J. S., & Breier, A. (1987a). The Vermont longitudinal study of persons with severe mental illness: I. Methodology, study sample and overall status 32 years later. *American Journal of Psychiatry, 144,* 718–726.

Harding, C. M., Brooks, G. W., Ashikaga, T., Strauss, J. S., & Breier, A. (1987b). The Vermont longitudinal study of persons with severe mental illness: II. Long-term outcome of subjects who retrospectively met DSM-III criteria for schizophrenia. *American Journal of Psychiatry, 144,* 727–735.

Hawkins, D.R. (1970). Implications of knowledge of sleep patterns in psychiatric conditions. In E. Hartmann (Ed.), *Sleep and Dreaming* (pp. 85–92). Boston: Little, Brown.

Hegarty, J. D., Baldessarini, R. J., Tohen, M., Waternaux, C. & Oepen, G. (1994). One hundred years of schizophrenia: A meta-analysis of the outcome literature. *American Journal of Psychiatry, 151,* 1409–1416.

Herz, M. J., Spitzer, R. L., Gibbon, M., Greenspan, K., & Reibel, S. (1974). Individual versus group aftercare treatment. *American Journal of Psychiatry, 131,* 808–812.

Hogarty, G. E. (1993). Prevention of relapse in chronic schizophrenic patients. *Journal of Clinical Psychiatry, 54*(3, Suppl.), 18–23.

Hogarty, G. E., Anderson, C. M., Reiss, D. J., Kornblith, S. J., Greenwald, D. P., Ulrich, R. F., Carter, M., & EPICS Research Group. (1991). Family psychoeducation, social skills training, and maintenance chemotherapy in the aftercare treatment of schizophrenia. II: Two-year effects of a controlled study on relapse and adjustment. *Archives of General Psychiatry, 48,* 340–347.

Hogarty, G. E., Anderson, C. M., Reiss, D. J., Kornblith, S. J., Greenwald, D. P., Javna, C. P., Madonia, M. J., & EPICS Research Group. (1986). Family psychoeducation, social skills training, and maintenance chemotherapy in the aftercare treatment of schizophrenia, I: One-year effects of a controlled study on relapse and expressed emotion. *Archives of General Psychiatry, 43,* 633–642.

Hogarty, G. E., Reiss, D. J., & Anderson, C. M. (1990). Psychoeducational family management of schizophrenia. In M. J. Herz, S. J. Keith, & J. P. Docherty (Eds.), *Handbook of Schizophrenia: Psychosocial Treatment of Schizophrenia* (Vol. 4, pp. 153–166). New York: Elsevier.

Hooley, J. M., Orley, J., & Teasdale, J. D. (1986). Levels of expressed emotion and relapse in depressed patients. *British Journal of Psychiatry, 148,* 642–647.

Horwath, E., Johnson, J., Klerman, G. L., & Weissman, M. M. (1992). Depressive symptoms as relative and attributable risk factors for first-onset major depression. *Archives of General Psychiatry, 49,* 817–823.

Horwitz, L. (1983). Projective identification in dyads and groups. *International Journal of Group Psychotherapy, 33,* 259–279.

Horwitz, L. (1994). Depth of transference in groups. *International Journal of Group Psychotherapy, 44,* 271–290.

Howe, C. W., & Howe, J. W. (1987). The national alliance for the mentally ill: History and ideology. In A. B. Hatfield (Ed.), *Families of the Mentally Ill: Meeting the Challenges. New Directions for Mental Health Services* (No. 34, pp. 23–33). San Francisco: Jossey-Bass.

Hulse, W. C. (1958). Psychotherapy with ambulatory schizophrenic patients in mixed analytic groups. *Archives of Neurology and Psychiatry, 79,* 681–687.

Jacobs, H. E., Wissusik, D., Collier, R., Stackman, D., & Burkeman, D. (1992).

Correlations between psychiatric disabilities and vocational outcome. *Hospital and Community Psychiatry, 43,* 365–369.

Janecek, J., & Mandel, A. (1965). The combined use of group and pharmacotherapy by collaborative therapists. *Comprehensive Psychiatry, 6,* 35–40.

Johnson, D., & Howenstine, R. (1982). Revitalizing an ailing group psychotherapy program. *Psychiatry, 45,* 138–146.

Johnson, H. (1992). *Sleepwalking Through History.* New York: Anchor Books/Doubleday.

Joint Commission on Mental Illness and Health. (1961). *Final Report of the Commission: Action for Mental Health.* New York: Basic Books.

Jones, M. (1948). Emotional catharsis and re-education in the neuroses with the help of group methods. In K. R. MacKenzie (Ed.), *Classics in Group Psychotherapy* (pp. 88–94). New York: Guilford Press, 1992.

Kanas N. (1985). Inpatient and outpatient group therapy for schizophrenic patients. *American Journal of Psychotherapy, 39,* 431–439.

Kanas, N. (1991). Group therapy with schizophrenic patients: A short-term homogeneous approach. *International Journal of Group Psychotherapy, 41,* 33–48.

Kanas, N., Deri, J., Ketter, T., & Fein, G. (1989a). Short-term outpatient therapy groups for schizophrenics. *International Journal of Group Psychotherapy, 39,* 517–522.

Kanas, N., & Smith, A. J. (1990). Schizophrenic group process: A comparison and replication using the HIM-G. *Group, 14,* 246–252.

Kanas, N., Stewart, P., Deri, J., Ketter, T., & Haney, K. (1989b). Group process in short-term outpatient therapy groups for schizophrenics. *Group, 13,* 67–73.

Katz, A. H., & Bender, E. I. (1976). *The Strength in Us: Self-Help Groups in the Modern World.* New York: Franklin-Watts.

Katz, G. A. (1983). The non-interpretation of metaphors in psychiatric hospital groups. *International Journal of Group Psychotherapy, 33,* 56–68.

Keith, S. J., & Mathews, S. M. (1984). Schizophrenia: A review of psychosocial treatment strategies. In J. B. W. Williams & R. L. Spitzer (Eds.), *Psychotherapy Research: Where Are We and Where Should We Go?* (pp. 70–86). New York: Guilford Press.

Keller, M. B. & Hanks, D. L. (1994). The natural history and heterogeneity of depressive disorders: Implications for rational antidepressant therapy. *Journal of Clinical Psychiatry, 55*(9, Suppl. A), 25–31.

Keller, M. B., Lavori, P. W., Coryell, N., Andreasen, N. C., Endicott, J., Clayton, P., Klerman, G. L., & Hirshfeld, M. A. (1986b). Differential outcome of pure manic, mixed/cycling and pure depressive episodes in patients with bipolar illness. *Journal of the American Medical Association, 255,* 3138–3142.

Keller, M. B., Lavori, P. W., Mueller, T. I., Endicott, J., Coryell, W., Hirschfield, R. M. A., & Shea, T. (1992). Time to recovery, chronicity, and levels of psychopathology in major depression: A 5-year prospective follow-up of 431 subjects. *Archives of General Psychiatry, 49,* 809–816.

Keller, M. B., Lavori, P. W., Rice, J., Coryell, W., & Hirschfeld, R. M. A. (1986a). The persistent risk of chronicity in recurrent episodes of nonbipolar major depressive disorder: A prospective follow-up. *American Journal of Psychiatry,* *143,* 24–28.

Kennard, D. (1993). The first session—an apparent distraction. In D. Kennard, J. Roberts, & D. A. Winter (Eds.), *A Work Book of Group-Analytic Interventions* (pp. 21–28). London: Routledge.

Kernberg, O. F. (1975). *Borderline Conditions and Clinical Psychoanalysis.* New York: Jason Aronson.

Kibel, H. D. (1990). The inpatient psychotherapy group as a testing ground for theory. In B. E. Roth, W. N. Stone, & H. D. Kibel (Eds.), *The Difficult Patient in Group* (pp. 245–264). Madison, CT: International Universities Press.

Kimmel, L. H. (1991). The concept of elastic boundaries applied to group therapy with veterans over 60 years old. *Archives of Psychiatric Nursing, 5*(2), 91–98.

Klapman, J. W. (1951). Clinical practices of group psychotherapy with psychotics. *International Journal of Group Psychotherapy, 1,* 22–30.

Klein, E. B. (1977). Transference in training groups. *Journal of Personality and Social Systems, 1,* 53–63.

Klein, E. B. (1992). Contributions from social systems theory. In R. H. Klein, H. S. Bernard, & D. L. Singer (Eds.), *Handbook of Contemporary Group Psychotherapy* (pp. 87–123). Madison, CT: International Universities Press.

Klein, R. H., Hunter, D. E. K., & Brown, S. (1990). Long-term inpatient group psychotherapy. In B. E. Roth, W. N. Stone, & H.D. Kibel (Eds.), *The Difficult Patient in Group* (pp. 215–244). Madison, CT: International Universities Press.

Klerman, G. L., & Weissman, M. M. (1992). The course, morbidity and costs of depression. *Archives of General Psychiatry, 49,* 831–834.

Koenigsberg, H.W., & Handley, R. (1986). Expressed emotion: From predictive index to clinical construct. *American Journal of Psychiatry, 143,* 1361–1373.

Koenigsberg, H. W., Klausner, E., Pelino, D., Rosnick, P., & Campbell, R. (1993). Expressed emotion and glucose control in insulin-dependent diabetes mellitus. *American Journal of Psychiatry, 150,* 1114–1115.

Kohut, H. (1971). *The Analysis of the Self.* New York: International Universities Press.

Kohut, H. (1977). *The Restoration of the Self.* New York: International Universities Press.

Kohut, H. (1984). *How Does Analysis Cure?* Chicago: University of Chicago Press.

Koranyi, E. K. (1979). Morbidity and rate of undiagnosed physical illnesses in a psychiatric clinic population. *Archives of General Psychiatry, 36,* 414–419.

Kottgen, C., Sonnichsen, I., Mollenhauer, K., & Jurth, R. (1984). Group therapy with the families of schizophrenic patients: Results of the Hamburg Camberwell family interview study III. *International Journal of Family Psychiatry, 5,* 84–94.

Kramer, M., & Roth T. (1979). Dream in psychopathology. In B. B. Wolman (Ed.), *Handbook of Dreams: Research, Theories and Application* (pp. 361–387). New York: Van Nostrand Reinhold.

Kripke, D. F., & Robinson, D. (1985). Ten years with a lithium group. *McLean Hospital Journal, 10,* 1–11.

Krystal, H. (1974). The genetic development of affect and affect regression. *Annual of Psychoanalysis, 2,* 98–126.

Kuhlman, T. L. (1992). Unavoidable tragedies in Madison, Wisconsin: A third view. *Hospital and Community Psychiatry, 43,* 72–73.

Kuipers, L. (1979). Expressed emotion: A review. *British Journal of Social and Clinical Psychology, 18,* 237–243.

Kupfer, D. J., Frank, E., Perel, J. M., Cornes, C., Mallinger, A. G., Thase, M. E., McEachran, A. B., & Grochocinski, V. J. (1992). Five-year outcome for maintenance therapies in recurrent depression. *Archives of General Psychiatry, 49,* 769–773.

Lamb, H. R. (1984). Deinstitutionalization and the homeless mentally ill. *Hospital and Community Psychiatry, 35,* 899–907.

Leff, J. (1988). *Psychiatry around the Globe: A Transcultural View.* London: Gaskell.

Leff, J., Kuipers, L., Berkowitz, R., Eberlein-Vries, R., & Sturgeon, D. (1982). A controlled trial of social intervention in the families of schizophrenic patients. *British Journal of Psychiatry, 141,* 121–134.

Leff, J., Kuipers, L., Berkowitz, R., & Sturgeon, D. (1985). A controlled trial of social intervention in the families of schizophrenic patients: Two-year follow-up. *British Journal of Psychiatry, 146,* 594–600.

Lehman, A. F. (1983). The well-being of chronic mental patients: Assessing their quality of life. *Archives of General Psychiatry, 40,* 369–373.

Leithauser, B. (1990, January 14). Kasparov beats deep thought. *New York Times Magazine.*

Leshner, A. I. (1992). A new system of care for the homeless mentally ill. *Hospital and Community Psychiatry, 43,* 865.

Lesser, I. M., & Friedmann, C. T. H. (1980). Beyond medications: Group therapy for the chronic psychiatric patient. *International Journal of Group Psychotherapy, 30,* 187–199.

Levene, H. I., Patterson, V., Murphey, B. G., Overbeck, A. L., & Veach, T. L. (1970). The aftercare of schizophrenics: An evaluation of group and individual approaches. *Psychiatry Quarterly, 44,* 296–304.

Levin, D., Diamond, R., & Golstein, S. (1985). A study of alternating leadership for group psychotherapy in an aftercare clinic. *Perspectives in Psychiatric Care, 13,* 33–38.

Levinson, D. J., Darrow, C. M., Klein, E. B., Levinson, M. H., & KcKee, J. B. (1978). *Seasons of a Man's Life.* New York: Knopf.

Liberman, R. P., Mueser, K. T., & Wallace, C. J. (1986). Social skills training for schizophrenic individuals at risk for relapse. *American Journal of Psychiatry, 143,* 523–526.

Lieberman, M. A. (1990). A group therapist perspective on self-help groups. *International Journal of Group Psychotherapy, 40,* 251–278.

Lonergan, E. C. (1991). Keeping a group psychotherapy program alive and well within a psychiatric residency. *Group, 15,* 168–180.

Low, A. A. (1950). *Mental Health through Will Training.* Boston: Christopher Publishing House.

Macaskill, N. D. (1982). Therapeutic factors in group therapy with borderline patients. *International Journal of Group Psychotherapy, 32,* 61–73.

MacKenzie, K. R. (1974). Holding tea groups: A home visiting program for chronic schizophrenics. *Hospital and Community Psychiatry, 25,* 509–512.

MacKenzie, K. R. (1990). *Introduction to Time-Limited Group Psychotherapy.* Washington: American Psychiatric Press.

MacKenzie, K. R. (1994). The developing structure of the therapy group system. In H. S. Bernard & K. R. MacKenzie (Eds.), *Basics of Group Psychotherapy* (pp. 35–59). New York: Guilford Press.

Malm, U. (1982), The influence of group therapy on schizophrenia. *Acta Psychiatrica Scandanavica* (Suppl. 297), 1–65.

Masnik, R., Bucci, L., Isenberg, D., & Normand, W. (1971). "Coffee and . . . ": A way to treat the untreatable. *American Journal of Psychiatry, 128,* 164–167.

Massion, A. O., Warshaw, M. G., & Keller, M. B. (1993). Quality of life and psychiatric morbidity in panic disorder and generalized anxiety disorder. *American Journal of Psychiatry, 150,* 600–607.

McCarrick, A. K., Manderscheid, R. W., Bertolucci, D. E., Goldman, H., & Tessler, R. C. (1986). Chronic medical problems in the chronic mentally ill. *Hospital and Community Psychiatry, 37,* 289–291.

McCourt, W. F., Williams, A. F., & Schneider, L. (1971). Incidence of alcoholism in a state mental hospital population. *Quarterly Journal of Studies on Alcohol, 32,* 1085–1088.

McGee, T. F. (1980). Transition in the cotherapy dyad: To wait or not to wait. *Group, 4,* 65–71.

McGee, T. F. (1983). Long-term group psychotherapy with post-hospital patients. In L. Wolberg, & M. Aronson (Eds.), *Group and Family Therapy* (pp. 93- 106). New York: Brunner/Mazel.

McGlashan, T. H. (1988). A selective review of recent North American long-term follow-up studies of schizophrenia. *Schizophrenia Bulletin, 14,* 514–541.

McGlashan, T. H., Levy, S. T., & Carpenter, W. T. (1975). Integration and sealing over: Clinically distinct recovery styles from schizophrenia. *Archives of General Psychiatry, 32,* 1269–1272.

McIntosh, D., Stone, W. N., & Grace, M. (1991). The flexible boundaried group: Format, techniques, and patients' perceptions. *International Journal of Group Psychotherapy, 41,* 49–64.

Mechanic, D., & Aiken, L. H. (1987). Improving the care of patients with chronic mental illness. *New England Journal of Medicine, 317,* 1634–1638.

Michaels, R. (1980). Adulthood. In S. I. Greenspan & G. H. Pollock (Eds.), *The Course of Life. Psychoanalytic Contributions Toward Understanding Personality Development: Vol. III. Adulthood and the Aging Process* (pp. 25–34). Washington, DC: U.S. Department of Health and Human Services.

Minkoff, K. (1989). An integrated treatment model for dual diagnosis of psychosis and addiction. *Hospital and Community Psychiatry, 40,* 1031–1036.

Minkoff, K., & Stern, R. (1985). Paradoxes faced by residents being trained in the psychosocial treatment of people with chronic schizophrenia. *Hospital and Community Psychiatry, 36,* 859–864.

Misunis, R. J., Feist, B. J., Thorkelsson, J. G., & McAuley, L. (1990). Outpatient groups for chronic psychiatric patients. *Group, 14,* 111–120.

Mosher, L. R., & Keith, S. J. (1980). Psychosocial treatment: Individual, group, family and community support approaches. In *Special Report: Schizophrenia 1980* (DHHS Publication No. ADM-81-1064, pp. 127–156). Rockville, MD: Department of Health and Human Services, National Institute of Mental Health.

Nemiroff, R. A., & Colarusso, C. A. (1985). *The Race against Time.* New York: Plenum Press.

Newton, P. M. (1973). Social structure and process in psychotherapy: A socio-psychological analysis of transference, resistance and change. *International Journal of Psychiatry, 11,* 480–523.

Nierenberg, A. A. (1994). The treatment of severe depression: Is there an efficacy gap between SSRI and TCA antidepressant generations? *Journal of Clinical Psychiatry, 55*(9, Suppl. A), 55–59.

Novalis, P. N., Rojcewicz, S. J., Jr., & Peele, R. (1993). *Clinical Manual of Supportive Psychotherapy.* Washington, DC: American Psychiatric Press.

Nuechterlein, K. H., & Dawson, M. E. (1984). Information processing and attentional functioning in the developmental course of schizophrenic disorders. *Schizophrenia Bulletin, 10,* 160–203.

O'Brien, C. P., Hamm, K. B., Ray, B. A., Pierce, J. F., Luborsky, L., & Mintz, J. (1972). Group vs individual psychotherapy with schizophrenics. *Archives of General Psychiatry, 27,* 474–478.

Parloff, M. B., & Dies, R. R. (1977). Group psychotherapy outcome research: 1966–1975. *International Journal of Group Psychotherapy, 27,* 281–319.

Payne, S. B. (1965). Group methods in the pharmacotherapy of chronic psychotic patients. *Psychiatric Quarterly, 39,* 258–263.

Pepper, B., Kirschner, M. C., & Ryglewicz, H. (1981). The young adult chronic patient: Overview of a population. *Hospital and Community Psychiatry, 32,* 470–474.

Peters, T. J. & Waterman, R. H., Jr. (1982). *In Search of Excellence.* New York: Warner Books.

Polan, S., & Spark, I. (1950). Group psychotherapy of schizophrenics in an outpatient clinic. *American Journal of Orthopsychiatry, 20,* 382–396.

Prien, R. F., & Gelenberg, A. J. (1989). Alternatives to lithium for preventive treatment of bipolar disorder. *American Journal of Psychiatry, 146,* 840–848.

Purvis, S. A., & Miskimins, R. W. (1970). Effects of community follow-up on post-hospital adjustment of psychiatric patients. *Community Mental Health Journal, 6,* 374–382.

Racker, H. (1968). *Transference and Countertransference.* New York: International Universities Press.

Rada, R., Draper, E., & Daniels, R. S. (1964). A therapeutic waiting area experience for patients with chronic psychiatric illness. *Comprehensive Psychiatry, 5,* 191–192.

A Recovering Patient. (1986). "Can we talk? The schizophrenic patient in psychotherapy. *American Journal of Psychiatry, 143,* 68–70.

Redl, F. (1942). Group emotion and leadership. *Psychiatry, 5, 573–596.*

Reich, J. H., & Green, A. I. (1991). Effect of personality disorders on outcome of treatment. *Journal of Nervous and Mental Disease, 179,* 74–82.

Rice, A. K. (1969). Individual, group and intergroup processes. *Human Relations, 22,* 565–584.

Rice, C. A., & Rutan J. S. (1987). *Inpatient Group Psychotherapy.* New York: Macmillan.

Roca, R. P., Breakey, W. R., & Fischer, P. J. (1987). Medical care of chronic psychiatric outpatients. *Hospital and Community Psychiatry, 38,* 741–745.

Rodenhauser, P. (1989). Group psychotherapy and pharmacotherapy: Psychodynamic considerations. *International Journal of Group Psychotherapy, 39,* 445–456.

Rodenhauser, P., & Stone, W. N. (1993). Combining psychopharmacotherapy and group psychotherapy: Problems and advantages. *International Journal of Group Psychotherapy, 43,* 11–29.

Roller, B., & Nelson, V. (1993). Cotherapy. In H. I. Kaplan & B. J. Sadock (Eds.), *Comprehensive Group Psychotherapy* (3rd ed., pp. 304–312). Baltimore: Williams & Wilkins.

Roth, B. E. (1990). Countertransference and the group therapist's state of mind. In B. E. Roth, W. N. Stone, & H. D. Kibel (Eds.), *The Difficult Patient in Group: Group Psychotherapy with Borderline and Narcissistic Disorders,* (pp. 287–294). Madison, CT: International Universities Press.

Runions, J., & Prudo, R. (1983). Problem behaviors encountered by families living with a schizophrenic member. *Canadian Journal of Psychiatry, 28,* 382–386.

Rutan, J. S., & Alonso, A. (1980). Sequential cotherapy of groups for training and clinical care. *Group, 4,* 40–50.

Rutan, J. S., & Stone, W. N. (1993). *Psychodynamic Group Psychotherapy* (2nd ed.). New York: Guilford Press.

Safer, D. J. (1987). Substance abuse by young adult chronic patients. *Hospital and Community Psychiatry, 38,* 511–514.

Scheidlinger, S. (1974). On the concept of the mother–group. *International Journal of Group Psychotherapy, 24,* 417–428.

Scheidlinger, S. (1982). On scapegoating in group psychotherapy. *International Journal of Group Psychotherapy, 32,* 131–143.

Schinnar, A. P., Rothbard, A. B., Kanter, R., & Adams, K. (1990). Crossing state lines of chronic mental illness. *Hospital and Community Psychiatry, 41,* 756–760.

Seeman, M. V. (1981). Outpatient groups for schizophrenia—ensuring attendance. *Canadian Journal of Psychiatry, 26,* 32–37.

Shapiro, T., & Emde, R. N. (1992). General introduction. In T. Shapiro & R. N. Emde (Eds.), *Affect: Psychoanalytic Perspectives* (pp. IX–XIII). Madison, CT: International Universities Press.

Shattan, S. P., Dcamp, L., Fujii, E., Fross, G. G., & Wolff, R. J. (1966). Group treatment of conditionally discharged patients in a mental health clinic. *American Journal of Psychiatry, 122,* 798–805.

Shea, M. T., Pilkonis, P. A., Beckham, E., Collins, J. F., Elkin, I., Sotsky, S. M., & Docherty, J. P. (1990). Personality disorders and treatment outcome in the

NIMH treatment of depression collaborative research program. *American Journal of Psychiatry, 147,* 711–718.

Sheets, J. L., Prevost, J. A., & Reihman, J. (1982). Young adult chronic patients: Three hypothesized subgroups. *Hospital and Community Psychiatry, 33,* 197–203.

Singer, D. L., Astrachan, B. M., Gould, L. J., & Klein, E. B. (1975). Boundary management in psychological work with groups: Issues of task, role, structure, contract and accountability. *Journal of Applied Behavioral Science, 11,* 137–176.

Slater, P. E. (1966). *Microcosm: Structural, Psychological and Religious Evolution in Groups.* New York: Wiley.

Slavson, S. (1957). Are there group dynamics in therapy groups? *International Journal of Group Psychotherapy, 7,* 115–130.

Snyder, K. S., Wallace, C. J., Moe, K., & Liberman, R. P. (1994). Expressed emotion by residential care operators and residents' symptoms and quality of life. *Hospital and Community Psychiatry, 45,* 1141–1143.

Spitz, R. (1963). *The First Year of Life.* New York: International Universities Press.

Spotnitz, H. (1957). The borderline schizophrenic in group psychotherapy: The importance of individualization. *International Journal of Group Psychotherapy, 7,* 155–174.

Spring, B. J., & Ravdin, L. (1992). Cognitive remediation in schizophrenia: Should we attempt it? *Schizophrenia Bulletin, 18,* 15–20.

Steinglass, P. (1987). Psychoeducational family therapy for schizophrenia: A review essay. *Psychiatry, 50,* 14–23.

Stern, D. (1985). *The Interpersonal World of the Infant.* New York: Basic Books.

Stone, W. N. (1983). Some dynamics of children's participation in after-care groups. *International Journal of Group Psychotherapy, 33,* 333–348.

Stone, W. N. (1991). Treatment of the chronically mentally ill: An opportunity for the group therapist. *International Journal of Group Psychotherapy, 41,* 11–22.

Stone, W. N. (1992). The place of self-psychology in group psychotherapy: A status report. *International Journal of Group Psychotherapy, 42,* 335–350.

Stone, W. N. (1993a). Groups for chronically mentally ill patients. In A. Alonso & H. I. Swiller (Eds.), *Group Therapy in Clinical Practice* (pp. 71–91). Washington, DC: American Psychiatric Press.

Stone, W. N. (1993b). Group psychotherapy with the chronically mentally ill. In H. I. Kaplan & B. J. Sadock (Eds.), *Comprehensive Group Psychotherapy* (3rd ed., pp. 418–429). Baltimore: Williams & Wilkins.

Stone, W. N. (1995). Group therapy for seriously mentally ill patients in a managed care system. In K. R. MacKenzie (Ed.), *Effective Use of Group Therapy in Managed Care* (pp. 129–147). Washington, DC: American Psychiatric Press.

Stone, W. N., Rodenhauser, P., & Markert, R. J. (1991). Combining group psychotherapy and pharmacotherapy: A survey. *International Journal of Group Psychotherapy, 41,* 449–464.

Stone, W. N., & Rutan, J. S. (1984). Duration of treatment in group psychotherapy. *International Journal of Group Psychotherapy, 34,* 110–117.

Sullivan, H. S. (1953). *The Interpersonal Theory of Psychiatry.* New York: Norton.

Sullivan, H. S. (1970). *The Psychiatric Interview.* New York: Norton.

Swann, A. C. (1995). Mixed or dysphoric manic states: Psychopathology and treatment. *Journal of Clinical Psychiatry, 56*(Suppl. 3), 6–10.

Swiller, H. I. (1988). Alexitithymia: Treatment utilizing combined individual and group psychotherapy. *International Journal of Group Psychotherapy, 38,* 47–61.

Talmadge, M. (1959). Values of group interaction for discharged mental patients. *International Journal of Group Psychotherapy, 9,* 338–344.

Test, M. A., Knoedler, W. H., Allness, D. J., & Burke, S. S. (1985). Characteristics of young adults with schizophrenic disorders treated in the community. *Hospital and Community Psychiatry, 36,* 853–858.

Thase, M. G., & Howland, R. H. (1994). Refractory depression: Relevance of psychosocial factors and therapies. *Psychiatric Annals, 24,* 232–240.

Thornicroft, G., & Breakey, W. R. (1991). The COSTAR Programme. 1: Improving social networks of the long-term mentally ill. *British Journal of Psychiatry, 159,* 245–249.

Tohen, M., Waternaux, C. M., & Tsuang, M. T. (1990). Outcome in Mania: A 4-year prospective follow-up of 75 patients utilizing survival analysis. *Archives of General Psychiatry, 47,* 1106–1111.

Tsuang, D., & Coryell, W. (1993). An 8 year follow-up of patients with DSM-III-R psychotic depression, schizoaffective disorder and schizophrenia. *American Journal of Psychiatry, 150,* 1182–1188.

Tuckman, B.W. (1965). Developmental sequence in small groups. *Psychological Bulletin, 63,* 384–399.

U.S. General Accounting Office. (1988). *Homeless Mentally Ill: Problems and Options in Estimating Numbers and Trends.* Washington, DC: Author.

Vaughn, C. E., & Leff, J. P. (1976). The influence of family and social factors on the course of psychiatric illness. A comparison of schizophrenic and depressed neurotic patients. *British Journal of Psychiatry, 129,* 125–137.

Verhulst, J. (1991). The psychotherapy curriculum in the age of biological psychiatry. *Academic Psychiatry, 15*(3), 120–131.

Vokmar, F. R., Bacon, S., Shakir, S. A., & Pferrerbaum, A. (1981). Group therapy in the management of manic–depressive illness. *American Journal of Psychotherapy, 35,* 226–234.

Walker, E., & Lewine, R. J. (1990). Prediction of adult-onset schizophrenia from childhood home movies of the patients. *American Journal of Psychiatry, 147,* 1052–1056.

Warner, V., Weissman, M. M., Fendrich, M., Wickramaratne, P., & Moreau, D. (1992). The course of major depression in the offspring of depressed parents: Incidence, recurrence and recovery. *Archives of General Psychiatry, 49,* 795–801.

Wechsler, H. (1960). The self-help organization the mental health field: Recovery, Inc., a case study. *Journal of Nervous and Mental Disease, 130,* 297–314.

Weiner, M. F. (1988). Group therapy in a public sector psychiatric clinic. *International Journal of Group Psychotherapy, 38,* 355–365.

Weiner, M. F. (1992). Group therapy reduces medical and psychiatric hospitalization. *International Journal of Group Psychotherapy, 42*, 267–275.

Weiss, J. (1993). *How Psychotherapy Works: Process and Technique.* New York: Guilford Press.

Wells, K. B., Burnam, A., Rogers, W., Hays, R., & Camp, P. (1992). The course of depression in adult outpatients. *Archives of General Psychiatry, 49*, 788–794.

Westermeyer, J. F. Harrow, M., & Marengo, J. T. (1991). Risk of suicide in schizophrenia and other psychotic and nonpsychotic disorders. *Journal of Nervous and Mental Disease, 179*, 259–266.

Whitaker, D. S., & Lieberman, M. A. (1964). *Psychotherapy through the Group Process.* New York: Atherton Press.

Wiesel, E. (1991). *The Fifth Son.* New York: Warner Books.

Wilson, M. (1993). DSM-III and the transformation of American psychiatry: A history. *American Journal of Psychiatry, 150*, 399–410.

Winnicott, D. W. (1965). *The Maturational Process and the Facilitating Environment.* New York: International Universities Press.

Winston, A., Pinsker, H., & McCullough, L. (1986). A review of supportive therapy. *Hospital and Community Psychiatry, 37*, 1105–1114.

Wolf, A. (1968). Psychoanalysis in groups. In G. M. Gazda (Ed.), *Basic Approaches to Group Psychotherapy and Group Counseling* (pp. 80–108). Springfield, IL: Thomas.

World Health Organization. (1979). *Schizophrenia: An International Follow-up Study.* New York: Wiley.

Wulsin, L., Bachop, M., & Hoffman, D. (1988). Group therapy in manic–depressive illness. *American Journal of Psychotherapy, 42*, 263–271.

Yalom, I. D. (1966). A study of group therapy dropouts. *Archives of General Psychiatry, 14*, 393–414.

Yalom, I. D. (1970). *The Theory and Practice of Group Psychotherapy.* New York: Basic Books.

Yalom, I. D. (1985). *The Theory and Practice of Group Psychotherapy* (3rd ed.). New York: Basic Books.

Young, J., & Williams, C. L. (1988). Whom do mutual-help groups help? A typology of members. *Hospital and Community Psychiatry, 39*, 1178–1182.

Zaslav, M. R., & Kalb, R. D. (1989). Medicine as metaphor and medium in group psychotherapy with psychiatric patients. *International Journal of Group Psychotherapy, 39*, 457–468.

INDEX